CW00408579

BEATING BACK PAIN
WITHOUT PILLS,
INJECTIONS OR SURGERY
– The ProSport Physio Way

BEATING BACK PAIN WITHOUT PILLS, INJECTIONS OR SURGERY
– The ProSport Physio Way

Dave O'Sullivan

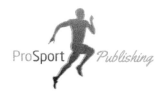

ProSport *Publishing*

ISBN: 978-1-674-74076-8

Copyright © 2019 David O'Sullivan

A CIP record for this book is available from the British Library

The moral right of the author has been asserted.

All rights reserved.

The Copyright Act prohibits (subject to certain very limited exceptions) the making of copies of any copyright work or of a substantial part of such a work, including the making of copies by photocopying or similar process. Written permission to make a copy or copies must therefore normally be obtained from the publisher in advance. It is advisable also to consult the publisher if in any doubt as to the legality of any copying which is to be undertaken.

Edited and typeset by Helen Jones

Facebook @BreathMoveHeal

Instagram @BreathMoveHeal

Twitter @BreathMoveHeal

This book is not intended as a substitute for the medical advice of physicians. The reader should regularly consult a physician in matters relating to his/her health and particularly with respect to any symptoms that may require diagnosis or medical attention.

Please note this book is written for the person living in pain and not medical professionals. There are times in this book where we simplify analogies and images and sacrifice 100% accuracy to help the everyday person understand key points with the best intentions to be honest and ethical so they can move forward and restore control of their bodies without getting confused and overwhelmed with medical terminology and the complexity of pain. Pain is a complex topic and it is beyond the scope of this book to be able to cover all the components of pain without overwhelming or confusing patients and hindering their ability to take action. The information outlined in this book is my current understanding, interpretation and opinion of the available evidence base to date in regards to low back pain.

Dedication

For Lily.

My inspiration and model for understanding 'perfect' movement when I was just starting out. Spending time with her and watching her allowed me a unique opportunity and insight to see how we should be moving effortlessly. Forever grateful.

You Don't Have To Do This Alone!

If you are living with back pain, then you are in the right place but there's no need to do this alone. I've created numerous tip sheets and recordings of some of the exercises to help you restore control of your body even quicker at **www.breathingmovinghealing.com**

Simply logon and download your tip sheets as well as an opportunity to join a safe and empowering Facebook community where we will do our best to answer all your questions.

Head over to **www.breathingmovinghealing.com** now for some great tip sheets and resources you can download free of charge.

Contents

Introduction

For Steve, one day things were going great. He was looking after his grandkids, going for long walks with his partner, waking to feel refreshed and ready for a day's gardening, and in general doing all the things he took for granted without a second thought. Then his pain suddenly started to affect all these things.

If you are like Steve or some of our other patients who initially came to ProSport Physiotherapy looking for help, you might have noticed a sharp stabbing pain or a constant dull ache that now consumes your attention instead of being able to spend time with family and friends uninterrupted...

You may notice first thing in the morning an unpleasant sensation of stiffness and pain in a body part.

You might even catch yourself holding your breath getting up and down off a chair or couch or picking something up.

You may notice you are standing differently and putting stress on other parts of your body which now may or may not be beginning to ache.

And some of our patients frequently admit to us that they were beginning to think the worst when the pain was at peak stages.

And worst of all, if you are like any of our patients that we successfully help on a daily basis, you might find yourself altering your lifestyle and not doing the things you enjoy doing with family and friends because of the pain, or worrying about paying for it later.

The common pitfall cycle of someone in pain

A few years back, we noticed here at ProSport Physiotherapy a common pitfall that patients tend to fall into.

You might have taken some paracetamol or even stronger painkillers and were told to rest from a well-meaning GP/Doctor. Initially this gives short-term relief but the pain sticks around and so you do some stretches you found on Google or that worked for a friend previously. Or perhaps you tried the exercise sheet from the NHS physiotherapy department after eventually getting an appointment after months of waiting but again it only offered very limited relief.

If you're anything like our patients who initially come to see us, you may have noticed the pain still hasn't shifted and is maybe actually getting worse and spreading to other parts of your body. Or other areas of the body have compensated and are becoming stiff now which may have you worrying about your long-term health.

And it goes without saying that it can also be worrying becoming more reliant on those anti-inflammatories and painkillers that may have an effect on your stomach and organs in the long term.

It's really sad to see when our patients tell us they have put daily activities, hobbies or activities aside or don't find them anywhere near as enjoyable as they once did. And for some people, this may affect their mood, energy and belief system about their long-term health.

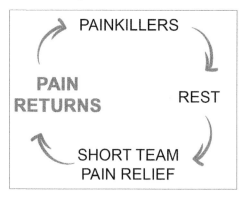

The common pitfall that we see happens to people before coming to see us at ProSport Physiotherapy. At ProSport Physiotherapy we strive to find the true cause and not just look at your symptoms.

At ProSport Physiotherapy, what makes us really different is We GET IT and UNDERSTAND this! Understanding the person in front of us ensures that you do not become just another 'patient' but we actually see YOU and WHAT YOU REALLY NEED to get the confidence back to doing things in your life that make you happy.

This book will help you move away from pain and towards building a happy, strong and resilient body that allows you to do the things in life that you enjoy most.

But first, a word of warning! This book is not a miracle cure with some gimmicky exercises that will allow you to momentarily touch your toes only for the changes to be short-term or give you a quick fix only for the pain to return with a vengeance later on. For most, recovering from persistent back pain (or any persistent pain) is not a linear process and there will be ups and downs and some challenges to your mindset. But what I can assure you is that if you are committed and want to move away from pain and towards a more resilient life then there is a natural way forward for you that has worked for many people in Huddersfield and surrounding areas.

If this way is so great, then why isn't everyone pain-free?

Well, there are three common mistakes I see people on a daily basis make when trying to overcome back pain that you need to know about and avoid if you too are to be successful.

MISTAKE 1 – FOCUSING YOUR ATTENTION ON THE SITE OF PAIN

You see, all those stretches, painkillers, ice and heat are focusing on the symptoms and never on the true problem specific to you. Just focusing on the area of pain is the equivalent of trying to lose weight by focusing all your attention on the scales, taking another layer of clothes off to try and influence the scales or trying to weigh yourself at different times of day to create small changes but never actually addressing the true problem which is usually all about diet and exercise.

Silly analogy, but hopefully you get the point. What is making your back, knee, shoulder, ankle or neck uncomfortable in the first place?

Now, stay with me with this explanation. It won't be as straightforward as this but, hopefully, this will help you understand why some people live in pain far longer than necessary.

Here's what SHOULD happen (give or take) when you bend down to pick something up, for example.

Now excuse my silly drawing but, as you go to pick your kids or grandkids up, the external load of their body weight plus your own body weight as gravity pushes you down need to be managed roughly in the following way.

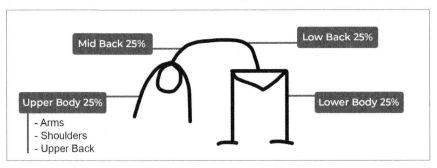

While we sacrifice a little accuracy for understanding here, you can see when we go to bend over or pick something up it's a whole body movement that needs the upper body, torso and lower body to all do their own job.

Your hands and arms will manage some of the body weight of the person you are lifting; let's say 25% for argument's sake. Your ribcage, muscles around your midsection and mid back will take 25% of that body weight, your low-back area may take 25% and your legs may take 25%, depending on the exact situation.

Now here's where it gets really interesting. Research has shown, and I've seen this consistently working in pro sport and serving thousands of people in Huddersfield for over 10 years now, that when we have had a previous injury, or there is weakness in an area or even a lot of stress in our lives, **our muscles REACT** and we form **new movement HABITS** to get through our day-to-day lives. The majority of times these new movement habits are so subtle we don't even notice them happening.

Think of a time when you may have rolled your ankle and you avoided putting weight through your big toe temporarily. Research has shown that the way we use the muscles all the way up to the hip can be slightly different for people who have had an ankle sprain.

So what's this got to do with your pain? Well, your brain is designed to protect you, first and foremost, and puts in these weird strategies short term to protect you from putting further stress on a body part. But if you take the stress away from one part of the body, usually you have to make up for that by putting more stress on another part of the body. These subtle new movement habits can NOW cause you to move with slightly different movement options. Let me demonstrate this with a few examples.

Here's what's happening for person A whose upper body, for whatever reason, is not doing enough (5%) so as you can see the mid back becomes slightly altered (down to 20%) and the low back now has to do more work as a result (50% instead of its usual 25%).

After a while, your low back tissues (muscles and nerves) may become 'a bit grumpy' and give your brain a signal that they are not quite happy doing the work of other body parts (50% instead of their usual 25%). That signal can often be pain or discomfort or your nerve may send a weird sensation down your leg. But I hope you can see that actually the low back is the HERO and doing a great job by doing the work of other areas of the body and it's the upper body in this case not doing its part. And I hope you can see that all those painkillers and back stretches will never actually address the true issue in this case – the upper body not contributing enough.

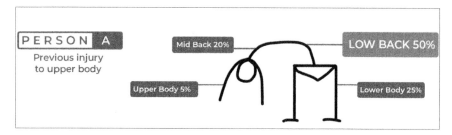

Here we see a person where the upper body is not doing enough work when lifting something and so the lower back area will have to work harder. In this person's case, the lower back is actually the hero and not the problem.

But here's the IMPORTANT SECRET. Person B has the exact same symptoms as Person A but they have had an old ankle injury in the past. You can see their lower legs aren't doing enough work (5% instead of 25%) and are causing the low back area to do more work (50%) with an adjustment in the rest of the mid back also (down from 25% to 20%) and the low back has to make up for the lack of work again.

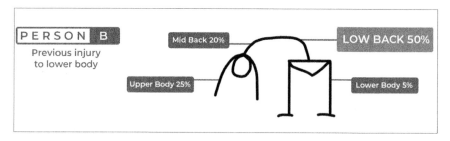

Although this person may appear to have the same symptoms as Person A, we see an old lower limb injury is causing their lower back to actually do more work than it might need to actually do. In this case, the lower back is the hero again but the true problem contributing to the pain sensation may actually need to be addressed in the lower body.

Another example might be Person C who has no previous injury but is having quite a stressful time at the moment; maybe he/she is not sleeping well and has had a big change in their lives recently. They find their mid back becomes stiff and is not doing enough (0%) so their low back does more work (50%).

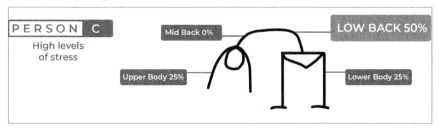

Here we see a person who may have had prolonged stress in their life recently or a traumatic event but not a previous big physical injury. When we have prolonged stress, we tend to breathe differently which may potentially affect how our mid back and ribs may function, which again may contribute to the lower back having to do more work.

Or in some cases, Person D who may have ALL of the above new habits and their low back is really fed up with doing all the work and taking up the slack, so to speak.

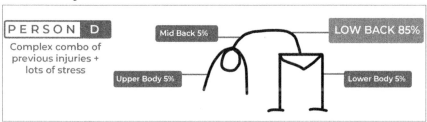

In some cases, it may be that a combination of physical and non-physical stressors are contributing to the person's lower back doing more work.

And we see the exact same thing happen with knee pain:

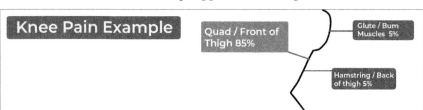

The front of the thigh muscles insert into the knee joint. These muscles sometimes have to do extra work with the knee joint to make up for the ankle and hip joints. Even though this person has knee pain, the true problem may be coming from the ankle or hip. The knee joint is again getting blamed unfairly.

And with shoulder pain:

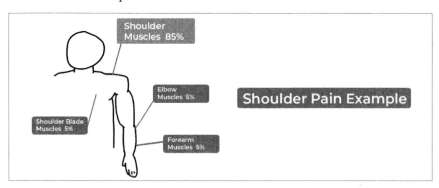

The shoulder joint may get unfair criticism for having to do more work for the wrist and elbow joint muscles and eventually ends up getting painful and weak. Although the shoulder is where the symptoms are, the true problem is the wrist and elbow joint muscles not doing their fair share of work.

So this is WHY IT'S ESSENTIAL WE UNDERSTAND YOUR STORY and make sense of the symptoms specific to YOU and don't just give you generic exercise sheets or painkillers but rather a movement plan that encourages ALL the parts of your body to work well together for long-lasting relief.

What about if I have been diagnosed with a known disc or nerve root issue?

While that is really beneficial to know, it still would not change our approach with your body. We would still want every other body part to do its job so the area around your disc or nerve root does not have to tolerate excessive load and potentially further sensitise that area. Think of the analogy of getting your thumb stuck in the door. You putting a plaster or padding over your thumb may help the pain levels short-term but if you keep banging your thumb with the door then it will probably continue to become even more sensitised. Our approach would be to take your thumb out of the door and allow your thumb to heal to the best of its ability while letting everything else do its job also.

Quick exercise for you

In the section below, list some of your previous injuries or possible stressful situations that may have caused you (or are still causing you) to breathe differently and possibly move differently:

1. _____

2. _____

3. _____

If you have seen other therapists in the past, have they looked at/or addressed any of these issues when dealing with your current pain?

1. Yes _____   2. No _____

This then leads us onto the second biggest MISTAKE.

MISTAKE 2 – A LACK OF CLARITY & UNDERSTANDING IN YOUR REHAB PLAN (OR JUST RELYING ON MASSAGE OR PASSIVE INTERVENTIONS)

A lot of the patients who come to us who have failed traditional approaches tell us they have seen other therapists in the past where they would lie on a massage bed for an hour or get their backs or joints manipulated once a week for a prolonged period and feel good leaving but then the pain would come back minutes, hours or days later.

And after the fancy drawings above, I hope you can start to see why this may only be a short-term pain relief strategy. The big mistake here is that there is little opportunity for your brain to develop the ability to work the TRUE problem area with the rest of your body once you've settled the symptoms down.

Many people spend hours doing, quite frankly, boring exercises like 'squeezing their glutes' or 'sucking the belly button in' or trying to 'keep the knee over the second toe' but the REALITY of LIFE is that **MOVEMENT is CHAOTIC in the real world** and you will not have time and should not need to think about your muscles doing all these things. It should happen automatically.

But most importantly **MOST OF THESE EXERCISES are NOT MEANINGFUL to your SITUATION and life.** It is essential that your movement plan is specific to your needs and not just random exercises with the hope that your brain will develop new movement habits.

The quickest, easiest and long-lasting way to develop different, non-painful movement habits is to show your brain the value of these movements and how much more efficient your movement is by doing it the way you once did when you were pain-free.

So, for a lot of our patients, it is just about reminding their brain of how they once moved and that is why our patients can enjoy changes in their pain sensation, stiffness and movement very quickly.

But, it's **NOT JUST ABOUT PAIN,** which leads me nicely to the final and **PROBABLY the BIGGEST REASON why people's pain keeps coming back…**

MISTAKE 3 – SKIPPING STEPS IN YOUR REHAB PLAN AND GOING BACK TO ACTIVITIES TOO SOON JUST BECAUSE THE PAIN IS GONE

I've seen this mistake being made so many times, even with pro sports athletes who come to see me who have failed traditional approaches – to return to the activities or sport that caused the pain, once the pain has eased, too soon. Instead you need to earn the right to progress to the next stage of your movement plan.

Imagine in my daily life of working with the Huddersfield Giants or England Rugby players and the day the pain eases doing a toe touch or some simple movement in the physio room, I'd just throw the player back out onto the field and into a chaotic rugby match situation. I don't think that would end very well and I'd probably lose my job.

Well, that's pretty much exactly what I see happening so often to people who were OK initially but the pain came back again. Most rehab exercises people are exposed to are too 'nice and controlled' like we touched upon in mistake 2.

If you look at the graph below you'll see most exercises the majority of people do in the physio room only stress our bodies a certain amount, at a certain speed of movement.

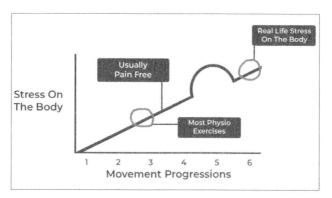

Most exercises done in the physio room may only stress your body a certain amount but in real life the stresses placed upon your body are actually much greater. This is why it's critical that we expose you gradually to the stresses of real life and ensure every part of your body does its own job, no more, no less, to give you the best chance of keeping the pain away long term.

But the biggest mistake I see is when a person's pain usually goes after, let's say, session 3 (see the graph below) and they try to jump straight back into the real world activities that happen at much greater stress and speed of movement than they were prepared for.

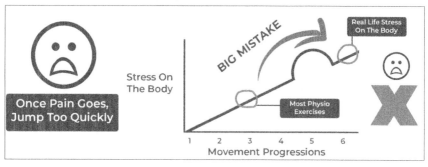

We need to expose our bodies to stress in a meaningful progressive way in order to build resilience to the stresses of daily life so that, when increased stresses are placed upon our body in the near future, we can cope with them rather than revert back to old habits.

In the real world, our bodies and brain need to be able to tolerate high levels of stress at different speeds. And unfortunately, most people are only exposed to nice slow and controlled movements in the physio clinic.

They skip steps, essentially, which is **WHY when they return to the real world, the brain may become overwhelmed and even frightened, perceive a threat to their safety and THEN REVERT BACK TO OLD MOVEMENT HABITS to survive.**

In the real world we don't have time to think about 'switching on muscles' as our kids are about to run out into the road and we reach and grab quickly, or we need to focus on something important and don't have time to think about 'squeezing our glutes' or 'sucking our belly button in'.

This is the real world and so we need to be prepared for that.

Which is why at Pro Sport Physio, **we don't GUESS you're ready to get back to your activities safely** without a big risk of the problem returning because **we don't skip steps in your movement plans.** We expose you to **MEANINGFUL MOVEMENTS** for you from day 1 and keep progressing you each session until you have genuine confidence to do the things you love doing with **THOUGHTLESS, FEARLESS MOVEMENT.**

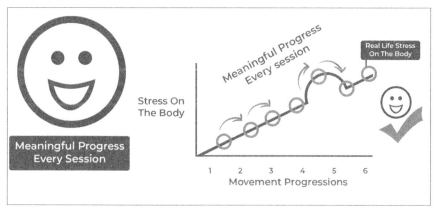

In this book you will learn how to build a solid foundation and earn the right to progress so you never skip steps and enjoy long-lasting results.

And when we follow the step-by-step plan which, by the way, is usually only a couple of sessions more after the pain eases, it **ACTUALLY SAVES YOU hundreds of pounds, sometimes even thousands in doctor's bills, physio bills, medication and in some cases even surgical bills.**

But, more importantly, it saves you time long-term and gives you back the ability to enjoy life with family and friends without your attention being consumed by pain.

So how do we ensure we do not make these same mistakes at ProSport Physiotherapy?

Here's what we have used over the past 10 years that has given us a 'go-to' therapist reputation in pro sport and private practice that has people travelling from all over Europe to visit our clinic for long-lasting results:

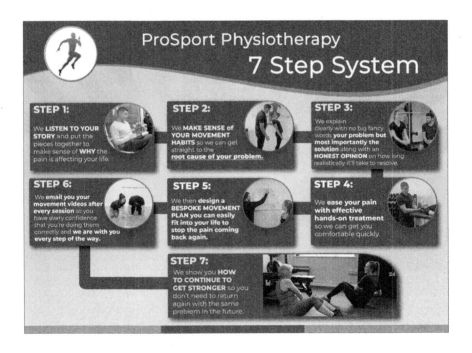

ProSport Physiotherapy

7 Step System

STEP 1:
We **LISTEN TO YOUR STORY** and put the pieces together to make sense of **WHY** the pain is affecting your life.

STEP 2:
We **MAKE SENSE of YOUR MOVEMENT HABITS** so we can get straight to the **root cause of your problem.**

STEP 3:
We explain clearly with no big fancy words **your problem but most importantly the solution** along with an **HONEST OPINION** on how long realistically it'll take to resolve.

STEP 6:
We **email you your movement videos after every session** so you have every confidence that you're doing them correctly and **we are with you every step of the way.**

STEP 5:
We then **design a BESPOKE MOVEMENT PLAN you can easily fit into your life** to stop the pain coming back again.

STEP 4:
We **ease your pain with effective hands-on treatment** so we can get you comfortable quickly.

STEP 7:
We show you **HOW TO CONTINUE TO GET STRONGER** so you don't need to return again with the same problem in the future.

STEP 1: We LISTEN TO YOUR STORY and put the pieces together to make sense of **WHY** the pain is affecting your life.

STEP 2: We **MAKE SENSE of YOUR MOVEMENT HABITS** so we can get straight to the **root cause of your problem.**

STEP 3: We explain clearly with no big fancy words **your problem but most importantly the solution** along with an **HONEST OPINION** on how long realistically it'll take to resolve.

STEP 4: We **ease your pain with effective hands-on treatment** so we can get you more comfortable quickly.

STEP 5: We then design a **BESPOKE MOVEMENT PLAN you can easily fit into your life to stop the pain coming back again.**

STEP 6: We **email you your movement videos after every session** so you have every confidence that you're doing them correctly and **we are with you every step of the way.**

STEP 7: We show you **HOW TO CONTINUE TO GET STRONGER** so you don't need to return again with the same problem in the future.

It's possible for you too

You too can live your day-to-day life without your attention being consumed with pain, medication or trips to consultants/doctors, exercises or stretches and you can give your family, friends and tasks your undivided attention once more.

You too can go on long walks, drives and flights without worrying about paying for it later and wake up the next morning ready to go again with that spring in your step and the confidence to enjoy your life to the fullest.

You too can have complete control of your physical independence and enjoy the future possibilities that life has to offer.

You too can wake up feeling great without a negative stabbing pain altering your mood.

You too can have the confidence to do those long outings without worrying if you'll pay for it later.

You'll feel lighter and springier...

You'll live life and play with your grandkids, spend time with your family and regain independence without relying on painkillers, GPs or other short-term fixes.

In this book I'm going to outline and teach you the exact steps we use here at ProSport Physiotherapy and also with professional athletes.

I'm going to teach you how to undo the major roadblocks that I see the majority of people in pain get stuck on so that you can improve your mood, energy and life.

Will you be completely pain-free by the end? That is impossible to say and anyone who says otherwise should be approached with caution. For some people, these movements will be enough; for others, they may notice a significant improvement in their pain levels, sleep and general energy, mood and lifestyle but may need a little more one-to-one help specific to their story. Remember everyone is different and will react differently to pain which is why sometimes you may need a different approach from the next person. But what you will get here is the best possible foundation and you will do the basics EXTRA-ordinarily so we give you the best possible chance before those final few steps specific to your needs are put into the treatment plan.

So now that the big issues are out of the way, let's get you started on your road to living free from pain and enjoying a happy, meaningful life.

I am going to be honest with you from the word go! The inspiration for writing this book was out of sheer frustration and disbelief at some of the things I was hearing from patients as they arrived through my door for their initial consultation with me. The majority of my cases these days are people who have had persistent pain despite a period of time passing where in theory the site of the injury should have been healed. The majority of these patients have 'seen everyone' and 'tried everything' to get rid of this pain. I am able to help the majority of these patients restore control of their own body (and mind) and they go on to live their lives pain-free.

I can help some patients restore control of their bodies and away from pain in four or five sessions, others it takes longer (6-8 sessions) and some a lot longer (12 sessions+). The biggest difference between patients that restore control of their bodies in four or five sessions versus the ones that take 12+ sessions from my own clinical experience is their 'beliefs' about their pain and acceptance of some of the information I am about to share with you in this book.

Back pain and sciatica are life-changing events if the pain persists. It is only until I ask some specific questions in my initial assessment with a patient that they actually stop, think about and realise the impact that back pain and sciatica has on their lives and the lives of their families and loved ones. Have a quick think about your answers to some of these questions below:

- Does your pain affect your ability to sleep through the night?
- Does your pain affect your first few steps in the morning when you get out of bed?
- Does your pain affect how you might move and bend down to reach for an object or lift something of moderate weight?
- When you do have to lift something of moderate load how does your breathing change?
- Do you find yourself holding your breath in anticipation or because of the pain?
- Do you find yourself avoiding or being reluctant to perform activities or tasks because of the 'price you'll pay later'?
- Does your pain affect your ability to help others with their lives – lifting your children or caring for your own parents, for example?
- Does your pain impact your mood?
- Does your pain bring feelings of anger, frustration or worry to your mind?

- Do you feel pessimistic or anxious about what your future life looks like?

The majority of patients will answer yes or be able to give some examples of how their pain affects their lives in relation to each of these questions above. The irony is that all these questions are interlinked and one answer may be contributing to you answering yes to another question. As you will learn in this book, everything in the human body affects everything else.

Let's look a bit closer at the impact of answering yes to the questions above or being able to give examples of how the pain is affecting your life.

Does your pain affect your ability to sleep through the night?

Sleep in my opinion is the most important area that we need to get right as it will give us the 'biggest bang for our buck' in restoring your ability to live pain-free. As you will see later, there is a big difference between how many hours sleep you get and the quality of your sleep and this is an important distinction that needs recognition.

Research has shown that your sleep can affect your pain levels as well as your mood, energy, food choices and even injury risk. Just think about a time when you didn't get much sleep – you were tired and fatigued the next day or days that followed, possibly. Your mood was a little bit more irritable than usual and you found yourself reaching for foods or drinks that you may not usually go for. A lack of good quality sleep causes massive changes in all systems in the body.

Those patients that come to my clinic with the most persistent pain look tired and fatigued, they lack colour in their faces, have a high breathing rate and complain that they haven't slept well in months. Intervening with and improving your sleep is one of the first things I will address with you in the clinic and in this book.

Does your pain affect your first few steps in the morning when you get out of bed?

Consider the implications of answering yes to the question above. Your first thought or sensation when you get out of bed is pain. How is that for a sensation to start every single day? What implications does this have on your mood starting the day in this way and how do your mood, energy and thoughts flow for the rest of that day?

Does your pain affect how you might move and bend down to reach for an object or lift something of moderate weight out of the car such as a baby?

Have you subtly changed how you now lift things of moderate weight or how you bend down to get that pen you dropped? Is getting up and down off the floor a challenge to you now? Should this really be how you move at your age? Is this how life will be from now on? Consider the implications of this on your life going forward.

When you do have to lift something of moderate load how does your breathing change?

Do you find yourself holding your breath or bracing even before you lift something of moderate load? Are you doing this automatically now in anticipation rather than a genuine need to brace? Consider the implications this has on your blood pressure, heart, arteries and veins. Again, is this normal for someone of your age?

Do you find yourself avoiding or being reluctant to perform activities or tasks because of the 'price you'll pay later'?

Is your pain or discomfort affecting your lifestyle choices and impacting you enjoying life to the full? Are you able to join friends for that long walk or hike? Are you able to ride your bike or play with your grandkids without their being a 'price to pay later' rather than the brilliant benefits and feelings you get from exercising and being active. Do you experience different feelings of pain, stiffness and worry?

Does your pain affect your ability to help others with their lives – lifting your children or caring for your own parents, for example?

Does the future require you to be in good health; will someone depend on you for help in the future? Will you be required to help your own children and look after your grandchildren in the future? Are your parents still alive and might they require support further down the line? Are the thoughts or feelings you get when you think of this in any way negative due to your pain levels?

Does your pain impact your mood?

Does your pain affect your relationship with others and your ability to engage in conversations or social events? Is this pain bringing a negative or a positive state of mind predominantly? Very often the pain will bring negative feelings and emotions which we will outline in more details later. Can you see how your pain can impact your state of mind and your ability to enjoy life to its full potential?

Does your pain bring feelings of anger, frustration or worry to your mind?

Do you feel anxious, worried, angry, frustrated, helpless or even depressed, or experience any other similar emotions at times due to your pain? If you answered yes, can you see how this is also impacting your state of mind? We will also discuss later how these feelings which may be completely unrelated to the pain at the time, may even trigger your pain.

Do you feel pessimistic or anxious about what your future life looks like?

Can you visualise yourself in 10 years' time enjoying a healthy, happy life without pain and having a healthy state of mind to go with it? This is very important to be aware of because usually the two go hand in hand as we will discuss later.

I hope you can see the value in stopping for a moment and thinking about the answers to the questions above and how they relate specifically to you and your life. Most people don't even realise how long their pain has been hanging around and the ACTUAL impact it is having on all aspects of their lives.

I do this exercise not to scare you into what lies ahead but to help you realise that enough is enough and now is the time to take action and change the answers to these questions. Now that you can see how your pain interlinks with your sleep, your breathing, your emotions, your movement behaviour and your general mood, it may come as no surprise that there is no magic exercise or 'manipulation' that will all of a sudden flick a switch, revert everything back to 'normal', whatever that is and give long-term meaningful change. I won't lie to you: it will take some commitment, work, determination, focus and effort but what I can say is that the rewards at the end will be worth it.

You will sleep through the night again and wake feeling refreshed, happy and raring to go and tackle the day ahead, jumping out of bed without experiencing any discomfort, stiffness or pain. Your first thoughts and feelings of the day will be positive rather than negative, painful sensations. You will move without thinking, bracing or holding your breath which will take excessive pressure off your heart, arteries and veins. You will get up and down off a chair or the floor without it feeling like an 'effort'. You will interact with friends and family without a second thought about the price you may have to pay later for enjoying the full benefits of life. You will help family members, friends and loved ones when they need help and you will have a healthy state of mind without the constant reminders and negative emotions that come with pain. You will enjoy all that life has to offer and have restored control of your own body.

Here's what to expect in this book which is broken down into three sections.

Section one helps you to change your belief system about everything we have spoken about up to now, to ensure that we put the foundations in place and you fully expect to achieve everything mentioned in the paragraph above.

Section two shows you how to apply the information you have learned in section one and really start taking action in getting to your destination, whatever that might look like.

Finally, section three is my tips, tricks and strategy section where I take you through a step-by-step guide to restoring control of your body using my tried-and-tested five-phase system.

If you can take one thing from this chapter without me being blatantly blunt about it up to now, it's this: this back pain or sciatica is no longer about your back. Your back is not the problem and never was the problem. I will explain more on this in later chapters. Now let's get to work and take that vitally important first step.

SECTION 1

Changing Your Belief System

CHAPTER 1

Can you really beat back pain and sciatica without pills, injections or surgery?

The simple answer to this question is yes. But to understand why I am so confident in answering yes so quickly, we first need to understand a little bit about what pain is. All pain is an OUTPUT of the brain. Now, before you think I am going to say that this pain is all in your head, I am not, so bear with me, please.

Pain is a very conscious sensation just like any other sensations. It is essentially an inbuilt alarm that you have designed to make you take action. Pain has been likened to a fire alarm going off in a building which could be caused by a guy smoking in the toilet or kids playing a prank. **IT DOES NOT MEAN DAMAGE nor if you do have a bulging disc or wear and tear around your low back that this is the entire extent of the problem.** It is a SIGN that your body wants you to change something. Possibly that how you are moving now is causing your low back and these areas where you do have wear and tear to be under excessive pressure. A pain sensation is essentially your subconscious mind 'PERCEIVING A THREAT' to your system and your body is POSSIBLY loading/using an area of the body too much and wants change or action.

The subconscious mind is influenced by messages coming up the spinal cord from the actual tissues (muscles, skin, fascia, ligaments and nerves) from your body and makes its decision whether to ignore these warning signals or send you a conscious experience of pain or discomfort.

Now it doesn't always need to be pain. If you are sitting in the same position for a long period of time such as on a car, plane or train journey, you might notice an unpleasant sensation around your bum and hip muscles and you may notice yourself moving around to try and get more comfortable. This would be an example where your body wants to change something or cause an action. This sensation is in part designed to achieve this. A conscious pain sensation may be a more extreme version.

Unfortunately you are not trained to find out exactly what your body is asking you to change, but this is where I come in, in helping you piece the clues together of your story. You see, YOUR PAIN sensation IS UNIQUE TO YOU. This is where there is no 'magic' exercise or an exercise that helped your next door neighbour's cat; your pain is influenced greatly by YOUR past history or your story as we like to call it. An ability to influence YOUR subconscious mind and reassure it that there is no actual threat, or possibly to change the movement HABITS you have become accustomed to, and give you greater options to move, can change the pain response quickly and dramatically if done in a correct manner. You are writing your own story at the moment and the great news about that is that you can change your story to whatever you want it to be. Your pain is INFLUENCED greatly by YOUR STORY and is unique to you. This is why a YOU-centered approach is essential and non-negotiable.

Your subconscious mind is ultimately concerned with keeping you safe. If you have conscious sensations of stress, anxiety or pain, it is letting you know it does not feel safe on some level. Why would YOUR subconscious mind think this? The answer to that question, outlined in further chapters, can help us greatly in piecing the parts of your story together to change the way you want to live your life.

And this information is great news for you because it means that when we change the OUTPUT of your brain by taking action in some very specific ways we will help you reassure your subconscious mind that the 'perceived threat' is not worthy of responding with such sensations as pain. Your life will be transformed, your mind will quieten from the constant pain signals it has been producing and you will enjoy life to the full.

I have seen many people just like you transform their lives and their family's lives by restoring control of their own bodies.

Pat, 65 (name changed to protect the patient's confidentiality) came to me with persistent low back pain that he had had for over 10 years. Pat was originally a builder but had to stop due to his inability to perform his duties. Pat is nearing retirement, has four grandchildren and has moved to the coast with his wife. Pat is a very quiet, unassuming man and was originally given my details by a mutual friend, Pat's brother. Pat had had another 'acute' relapse of back pain and his brother suggested he see me. Pat didn't do anything special; he just followed my instructions to the tee and performed the exercises that I recommended for him. No magic tricks or pills, just a little focus, determination and belief on both our parts.

I explained to him everything that I am going to share with you in this book, and over the course of six sessions Pat was free from living in pain. Pat had restored his ability to live life without pain. Pat's case was your typical case where we made some great gains quickly, had a few minor setbacks (such is life) and then went on to completely resolve the 'threat signals' that were responsible for the output of pain.

The final piece to Pat's puzzle was 'reassuring' his system that it was safe to put pressure through all parts of his left foot after he had sustained a bad ankle sprain years and years ago. Once we resolved and restored this ability, the last of Pat's pain sensation disappeared.

In Pat's case, his ankle and leg weren't doing enough work, so perhaps his low back was compensating. Once we got that percentage back up for his leg and ankle, his low back percentage was able to decrease and the pain sensation was finally able to go completely.

It was about six months later when a lady approached my wife and asked if she was married to me, which my wife confirmed. The lady asked my wife to thank me for what I had done for Pat. The lady was Pat's daughter who informed my wife that Pat was now like a completely different person, able to enjoy life again, able to listen to his wife and kids when they talked to him and actually able to interact and enjoy playing with his grandkids. Pat is now back working on a construction site part-time doing what he loves doing, on his terms.

This is the power of living life pain-free. You owe it to yourself to remember that feeling of living life pain-free and enjoying life again. I am with you every step of the way to show you the exact step-by-step process I went through with Pat and how to make it specific to you and your story.

CHAPTER 2

Why must you take action now and beat back pain and sciatica?

You must beat back pain and/or sciatica because you have the right to live pain-free regardless of events, circumstances or injuries that have happened to you previously. Once you start looking at the body as one big system, you may understand why your internal alarm is going off, regardless of what your X-ray or MRI report findings show.

Pain does not always mean damage

Pain is good at alerting us to take action but does not necessarily mean damage or that the wear and tear you have in your body is the complete cause of this pain sensation. I'd be a rich man if I had a pound for every rugby league player who came in and was going to collapse with pain in their foot, hand etc. and yet when the X-ray came back all clear, suddenly their pain levels dropped dramatically. The fear of the unknown is sometimes worse than reality. If there is a known mechanism or traumatic incident then this needs to be respected and can give us clues to the next step for you, yet for most people the pain is not a true indicator of actual damage to the body. Our bodies are very durable and our minds can heal and dampen down the pain very quickly if given the correct stimulus combined with education, understanding and even some hands-on treatment, if appropriate.

I am fortunate enough to work with rugby players who have wear and tear present on scans yet are completely pain-free and training and playing to an international level. Pain is not a good barometer for the reality, just like smoke alarms are not always accurate to the true level of threat present.

Your subconscious mind's priority is to keep you safe

Your subconscious mind is ultimately concerned with keeping you safe. It makes a PREDICTION of what MIGHT happen in the future but cannot actually predict what WILL happen. It controls the tone of the muscles (it actually sends that muscle spasm or tightness you may be feeling), your breathing rate, your heart rate and how you feel. It is mainly concerned with keeping you safe. You could ask yourself this: just before my pain or anxiety etc. started why would my subconscious mind feel the need to keep me safe and react like this? This can give you some clues. Influencing your subconscious mind to change your habits can be tricky but by the end of this book you will have the skill-sets and the understanding of how the body works as one and how ultimately we need to change your subconscious mind's PERCEPTION. We do this via breathing, exercise and even hands-on treatment, if required. We understand we need to change habits and help guide you to allow your body to heal just as it is designed to do.

How does pain originate?

Our tissues contain special messengers that are called 'nociceptors' that send a signal to the brain letting it know they are feeling a little irritated. The brain will then decide if this is a serious threat and IS REALLY DANGEROUS or just an overreaction from these messengers. These 'nociceptors' are sending signals to the brain all the time and in most cases the brain does not take action. The brain may choose to act and send a small sensation into your conscious awareness in the form of a small ache, for example. This may result in you taking action after a while and shuffling in your seat or moving around a little 'to get comfortable'. You have taken action when it suited you and the stimulus is no longer present.

The other option is that the brain can also really crank up the sensation you feel in the form of intense, sharp shooting pains that are essentially designed to stop you in your tracks and take action RIGHT NOW. When the messengers' signals persist, the SENSITIVITY of the messages increases to the brain and the brain may take notice a lot more easily than before so that even smaller movements that 'used not to hurt' now hurt, or pain is triggered even when moving other parts of the body. This can cause the brain to send pain signals even quicker yet there is ACTUALLY no change in the amount of wear and tear on your body.

Think about it – have you ever been in absolute 10 out of 10 agony and then five minutes later the pain quietens to a 4 out of 10? Not a whole lot internally around your low back may have changed in those five minutes.

The level of pain is influenced by other factors as well as the messengers' signals such as context of the pain, your own beliefs or thoughts about what MIGHT be wrong, where you are actually situated/your environment and previous experiences – these are all important to consider. This may give you clues why your pain becomes worse in certain environments or even when you are around a certain somebody. Your subconscious may be associating this place or thing with a past experience that may be contributing to your subconscious mind 'feeling' unsafe. Your subconscious mind takes into consideration your conscious beliefs about what the pain might be, and your context, environment and past experiences when deciding how intense the pain signal should be.

I have noticed a VICIOUS FORMULA amongst people with persistent pain that must be disrupted at all costs!

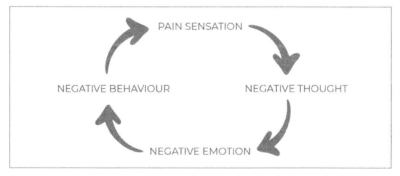

For example, you get a pain sensation around your lower back ⇨ THOUGHT – 'Oh no! My back is fragile and needs to be protected'; or in an extreme case 'My neighbour down the road had a bad back and is now in a wheelchair, I must be really careful with my back and protect it at all costs' ⇨ EMOTION – Scared, frightened, angry, anxious ⇨ BEHAVIOUR – Move in a slow, rigid, careful manner holding your breath in anticipation of pain appearing in the low back region.

The ironic thing about this is when you move in a slow rigid manner while holding your breath you actually put even more load and work on the back which further increases the communication from the low back to the brain. When we move in a relaxed manner and allow our mid back, legs and arms to contribute and move as one, we decrease the load on the low back, we decrease and interrupt the signals from the low back to the brain and we start forming new movement habits or remind our brain of how we used to move prior to this new movement strategy.

So you see, if you don't take action then the pain signals will more than likely continue to be sensitised and continue to be present until you take action and form new movement habits. So you really do need to take action now before the nociceptors become further sensitised and it takes even longer to desensitise them. The hardest step is the first step so you really need to take action now.

This is why education is the first step and you are taking that right now by reading this book. Education is so important because it helps you understand what pain REALLY is and what it isn't. It is not all about DAMAGE to a particular tissue.

The aim of this book is to empower you with education, hands-on treatment, exercise therapy and movement possibilities to restore the options available for your brain.

I appreciate taking that first step is scary but my team and I are here every step of the way and we have a supportive community to help you at **www.breathingmovinghealing.com**. Go there now and join our special Facebook group where you can meet others going through this journey.

CHAPTER 3
Why has low back pain and sciatica been so confusing up to now?

Low back pain and sciatica was confusing to me, and in some ways it still is. Good teachers are always learning. It used to bother me that low back pain and sciatica was so confusing, but once I found out what I'm about to share with you, I began to realise that I wasn't as much to blame as were the media, websites and blogs out there that have in essence misinterpreted a lot of the research done on the human body.

Low back pain and sciatica can be confusing because PAIN CAN CONTINUE EVEN WHEN TISSUES HEAL. From working in pro sport, I can tell you first-hand that tissues can heal very quickly. And most tissues will heal within 12 weeks if there is a known mechanism of injury, certainly enough to allow you to function sufficiently during daily life. However, sometimes the pain signals can persist even when the tissues have healed. The constant or repetitive communication between the nociceptors and the brain means the brain has become much more SENSITIVE to these messengers and continues to do what it did before by sending a conscious awareness of pain when these messengers communicate with it. This means that the messengers might now only have to whisper and the brain will send the same pain levels as before when the messengers had to really shout from the rooftops before the brain sent the pain signals. So now the EXACT same movements that gave you pain initially, still give you pain. Sometimes even less load can do the same. This can cause you to 'guard' certain movements and 'believe' that certain movements are dangerous when in fact it is actually those messengers' relationship with the brain which has become too close and the brain now trusts EVERYTHING the messengers say.

Remember: anytime we move with guarded movement, we more than likely increase the % contribution of the low back area and it ends up doing far more work than the 25% (give or take) it's meant to do.

One of the biggest misinterpretations of the research is the 'pulling or sucking your belly button in' myth before you perform an exercise or activity. All this research was based on the findings that the transverse abdominis muscles had a slightly delayed activation in people with back pain than those without. This transverse abdominis muscle is a 'corset-like' layer of muscle that surrounds the inner spine. One way that clinicians attempt to isolate this muscle is to have you 'suck your belly button in'. This research gained enormous popularity and even made its way into the fitness world with trainers recommending that clients tuck their belly buttons in when performing exercises. The reality of the situation is that the transverse abdominis muscle is only one small muscle out of a number of muscles that REACTS to pain. Attempting to isolate this muscle is non-meaningful because it needs to work as part of a team of muscles to help stabilise the spine. In section three, I will teach you how to 'activate' this muscle subconsciously, in a much more meaningful way for your brain, along with a number of other key spinal stabiliser muscles, without having to think about 'tucking or sucking your belly button in'.

The next misinterpretation I see in the literature is the notion of the 'glute muscles switching off'. Admittedly, I used to interpret the research like this in my early career, although thankfully I have seen the light and now use faster ways to engage these muscles in much more meaningful movements which I will share with you below. What has been shown in the literature is that when 'nociception' (messengers to the brain that contribute to pain output) are sensitised, or there is pain, the system chooses to avoid putting pressure on this area if at all possible (think spraining your ankle and limping for a few days). The muscle itself is still working just fine but it appears that certain motor units within that muscle synapse with the nociceptors and can cause these to alter the output with regards to the timing of an activity and the amount of activity IN A CERTAIN DIRECTION. Your body is very clever, however, and puts in alternative strategies (just like limping) very quickly to get the task at hand done. The problem is that many clinicians have interpreted this information as needing to isolate the whole muscle to 'activate' it. The muscle can recruit just fine as a whole – it is just certain motor units in certain directions that need reassurance. These motor units such as those in the foot, knee, back, shoulder, elbow and wrist need to work well with the rest of the body in order for you to be successful in life. Therefore, isolating muscles in NON-MEANINGFUL ways may be of limited benefit and, from my own experience of using these methods earlier in my career, time-consuming and not long-lasting.

Remember we want the upper body to do 25% (give or take) of the work, the mid back to do 25%, the low back to do 25% and the lower body to do 25%: nothing more, nothing less. We just want every body part to do its job.

What I have done in this book is to explain the interaction between the key systems of the body and how we can easily integrate all these systems together for you to reassure your nervous system of any potential 'perceived threats' and restore your movement options to address your altered movement behaviour and other factors mentioned previously.

CHAPTER 4

What will your life be like after low back pain and sciatica?

Now this might seem like a strange chapter title but I think it's very important to address this topic now and just take a moment to think about what your life will look like after your back pain is eliminated.

Now while this is absolutely not the case for the vast majority of people, for a small minority, their back pain may actually represent a safety blanket to avoid them being exposed to potential harmful situations or environments. For example, for some people, having persistent back pain may mean that they do not have to return to a job they hate or avoid working with a person they dislike. So actually, on some subconscious level, their current low back pain is actually protecting them from what their subconscious mind may perceive as an even greater threat.

Now while this isn't the case with the majority of people we see here at the clinic, it is worth thinking about the simple question below:

'Are there any advantages in my present situation to having back pain?'

Does it mean I don't have to go to an environment I don't particularly enjoy, see a person I absolutely dread with fear? Does it change your relationship with a certain somebody?

Again, while I do not want to go too left field, I still think it's important to consider this question and ask is there any reason your subconscious mind may choose to give you this conscious unpleasant sensation in an effort to protect you from something that may hurt you more?

If the answer is yes, it's OK. Nothing needs to be done with this information right now and I would encourage you to continue through with this book but it's just useful to start connecting the dots of how other factors may also contribute to your pain sensation. It may or may not need addressing further down the line but it is still very useful to be aware of now so that you can begin to process this information.

So now that this particularly awkward question is out of the way and you are 100% ready to live free from pain and enjoy life to the fullest, let's proceed to the next chapter.

CHAPTER 5

If pain is a conscious sensation, what actually is low back pain and sciatica pain then?

OK, so now you've gained an appreciation of the pain process, this does not mean that we need to completely neglect the low back or buttock region. The low back area and the muscles around the sciatic nerve will have some alterations in some of the motor unit's timings and resting tone.

If the sciatic nerve is genuinely involved, then it can be sensitised (think your thumb getting trapped in the doorway). You might just brush your thumb up against something lightly a day or so later but it still hurts because it's sensitive from the original issue of getting trapped in the door. Nerves can act like this and, from my experience, take a little longer to settle down than if they are not sensitised and are not a major contributor to the back pain episode.

Our approach in this book doesn't change even if you have a sensitised nerve or are diagnosed with a bulging disc. We take excessive load off the low back where the nerve originates and we get everything else doing its job so we give the nerve the best chance to heal and desensitise or the disc has an opportunity to reabsorb. Relearning how to move in a relaxed energy-efficient manner is the best way to mobilise your nerves, from my experience, working as part of one big team.

Some of the muscles in the low back area and gluteal area may be carrying some protective tone and may not want to produce a motor output when the body is in certain positions or moving in certain directions and you may be subconsciously avoiding these positions.

The ideal movement strategy consists of using the right amount of energy appropriate to get the job done. The problem is when there is a 'perceived threat' or 'pain' – parts of the muscle may have lost the ability to produce force suboptimally at low forces, which is important for everyday tasks, and may be required to work at maximal levels only recruiting the big fast twitch fibres instead of the slow twitch oxidative fibres for the majority of the day. The problem with this is that the bigger fast twitch fibres fatigue easily while the slow twitch oxidative tissues are more fatigue-resistant and essential to recruit for movement efficiency. Said another way, your body may be using far too much energy to do a simple task that actually only requires half the amount of energy. This can be an exhausting experience for a lot of patients in pain.

ACTIVITY

Take a moment to notice how you are sitting right now.

Feel the muscles that run along your low back, parallel to your spine.

Are those muscles taut and working hard?

For a lot of people these muscles will be working very hard all day long, even in supposedly relaxing activities such as sitting.

Now make a fist with your hand and fingers and squeeze your fist as tightly as possible.

After 30+ seconds or so, your muscles may start to ache; your wrist and fingers may even become painful.

This is what the low back muscles are doing 24/7 for a lot of people in pain. They are constantly working very hard.

What is the easiest way to stop your fingers and wrist aching? To relax your fingers right?

And so the quickest way to allow the low back from aching is to relax the low back.

However this is easier said than done. It is far more difficult to relax than it is to tense.

In the coming chapters I will show you some very useful tips to allow our low backs to relax and decrease the pain sensation.

Imagine keeping your fingers tense but opening your fist and trying to pick up a cup of tea with fully tense fingers. The movement would be jerky, slow and probably not well-coordinated just like the way we move when we have low back pain, in a very slow, rigid manner.

It is our job to reassure the system that it is now safe for these muscles to contract and relax in an energy-efficient manner in particular directions. I hope you can now see the importance of making sure the muscles are doing their own jobs and not working too hard.

First, we have to set up a good foundation where oxygen is travelling throughout the body more efficiently and you are using your diaphragm and pelvic floor to the best of their ability. Then we need to update your subconscious mind's belief system with meaningful movements and tasks to ensure it feels safe in positions that it may have previously avoided or coped with by using high threshold strategies. Not only this, but we need to change any altered or protective postures or breathing strategies you may have become accustomed to using, to ensure your body feels safe and can truly update its belief systems.

Once we get these basics mastered for the three fundamental movements that we use every day, it is time to add some load in a graded exposure so that your body can now tolerate additional loading without reverting into protective strategies once more. This is a fine balancing act and needs to be done systematically using my five-phase approach to ensure we always keep going forwards and do not plateau or progress too soon.

Now, all this might look a bit of a simple approach, especially if you have been unsuccessful with prior approaches but remember 'genius demands simplicity'. We are not trying to turn you into something you are not or making any wild claims about what we are doing here. We are simply

RESTORING the ability of your system and its sub-systems to function as they once did, to a time when you had no pain and plenty of movement options and everything doing its own job – nothing more, nothing less.

Once you understand the basics in chapters 9 and 10, you can then effortlessly integrate the major systems of the body to work together efficiently and easily for any injury you have during your life. I will be walking you through this in minute detail and am with you every step of the way.

SECTION 2

Getting Ready

CHAPTER 6

What are you really going to need to do to eliminate low back pain and sciatica?

OK, so now let's talk about the 'Beat Back Pain and Sciatica without Pills, Injections or Surgery Preparation Toolkit' that you will require for this programme to be effective. I hope you're ready and have your shopping list to hand. Here is what you require for this programme:

Physical requirements:

- Your nose
- Your tongue
- Your brain
- Your feet
- Your hands
- Two balloons

Mental requirements:

- A deep motivation to get back to living life pain-free
- A belief that you can live pain-free again
- An open mind
- An acceptance that it may be a week, two weeks, three weeks before you begin to notice changes
- Pig-headed determination and discipline to keep going with the programme
- An acceptance that your pain levels may vary and even rise initially
- A mindset that is ready for the implications of not living in pain anymore.

Physical requirements explained

We don't need any fancy equipment to help us restore what we once had. We only need our nose for breathing, our tongue for correct positioning to help our airway function correctly, our brain to stimulate the cranial nerves with some simple drills and our hands and feet to help us move and perform meaningful tasks. The two balloons will be used in exercises to help your breathing which I will explain in chapter 9. That is all I need to help a patient restore control of their own bodies.

In the clinic setting, I will also use my own hands if I feel your tissues may need some 'non-threatening' stimulus and I also may occasionally use a heart rate variability monitor with patients to get an exact insight of when is the best time to perform the restoration programme.

Mental requirements explained

The mental requirement is slightly more demanding yet very realistic as very often I find that once we start some breathing desensitisation drills then the self-doubt, anxiety, worry, negative voices and pain levels quieten down anyway. Therefore the hardest step is well and truly taking action and starting this programme. Motivation is absolutely essential and your motivation should not simply be 'to not live in pain anymore'. You need a deep motivation to return to some meaningful tasks or activities that you LOVE doing and WANT to get back to. Those are your motivating factors, not to get out of pain. Your subconscious mind cannot process negatives, therefore don't tell your subconscious what you DON'T want but tell it actually what you do want and where you want to be and let it go about getting you there.

You also require an open mind with some of the exercises and trust that they are helping you even if you cannot sense a change immediately. Remember, we are changing movement, breathing and mindset habits and, unfortunately, to achieve long-lasting results this takes time; every person responds at their own pace and that is fine. You will require determination to keep going through the times when you cannot feel a major difference but your motivation of the tasks you want to get back to should be so strong that your determination takes care of itself. Finally, you need to understand and accept the pain process and that if your pain levels do increase at any stage this does not mean you are causing yourself further damage but rather that the 'system' is sensing a change and is simply not yet convinced. In this scenario, we may have pushed too quickly or we may need to be even better at doing the basics EXTRA-ordinarily.

CHAPTER 7

What does the 'Beat Back Pain and Sciatica without Pills, Injections or Surgery System' involve?

The 'Beat Back Pain and Sciatica without Pills, Injections or Surgery System' involves five key phases and some sub-systems within each stage in order to progressively restore control of your body and mind without causing further protective tone or sensations, from my clinical experience. The system is set out to help you get the most bang for your buck and to help you get the foundations in place first and foremost before we get to any fancy exercises.

PHASE 1: Restore control of your thoughts

The first phase is to stop this vicious cycle that happens when we experience pain: Thought ⇨ Emotion ⇨ Behaviour.

We need to restore control of our thoughts and not allow them to feed forward into negative emotions that compromise our behaviour. The first thing we will do is focus your subconscious mind on where you want to get back to and give your subconscious mind a destination to work towards, very much like a GPS. If we were in a car in London, we would not set a GPS to get to Huddersfield by saying 'anywhere but London'. The chances of arriving at my doorstep in Huddersfield would be slim or next to none. Similar we do not tell our subconscious mind that we just 'don't want to have back pain'. We need to be very specific and intentional in how we want to feel again to give our subconscious mind a destination to work towards. The clearer the instructions for the subconscious mind (a full postcode to my home address), the greater the chance we give ourselves to arrive at this destination.

I will talk you through a very specific exercise for this and we will use this image to interrupt the cycle of pain ⇨ negative thoughts ⇨ negative emotions ⇨ deconstructive behaviour.

PHASE 2: Restore control of the respiratory system

The second phase in the 'Beat Back Pain and Sciatica without Pills, Injections or Surgery System' is restoring control of your respiratory system. The majority of people in pain hold their breath when they perform certain movements in anticipation of pain before it might even occur. This, along with the emotions and feelings that come with pain, causes the person to often have an increased breathing rate (the amount of breaths you take per minute) and also an increased volume of breath (the amount of air you take in per breath). Taking more air in is not advantageous as we can only use a certain amount of oxygen per breath and deliver it around the body. We therefore avoid overworking many muscles in the body and get two key pumps of the body, the diaphragm and pelvic floor working well together again. We will restore the lengthening ability of these muscles and desensitise the need to breath at increased rates and depths.

An added benefit is this helps to quieten your mind and impacts phase 1 further, allowing you to match your breathing to that of 'rest and digest' and change the constant 'fight or flight' autonomic system dominance. Not only this but it will improve the quality of your sleep, improve the peripheral and spinal muscles' delivery of oxygen and help decrease the stiffness and achiness of the muscles. Performing these simple exercises before bed has helped a lot of my patients to sleep better and they wake up feeling refreshed and energised; this will obviously have an impact on your mood.

The final and most important benefit of addressing this is that we improve the function of the diaphragm and pelvic floor by reducing protective tone. These two muscles are ESSENTIAL core muscles that are very often overlooked. If we cannot lengthen our diaphragm then the ability of the transverse abdominis muscle is straight away compromised (don't even worry about sucking your belly button in) and if we cannot shorten our pelvic floor, then the gluteal muscles will have an altered length tension relationship when the pelvis posteriorly tilts. I hope you can see the advantage of getting this stage correct before moving onto stages that the majority of therapists will start with when the foundations are not in place yet.

PHASE 3: Restoring a relaxed low back while sitting and standing

The third phase is addressing the biggest problems first. Rather than giving you three sets of 10 of certain exercises, we are going to address the big activities that you spend hours doing every day – sitting, getting up and down off a chair and standing. If we can allow your low back to do 25% of the workload in all these activities and get everything else to do their jobs along with restoring control of your thoughts and restoring a more efficient respiratory system, then by this stage you may notice some positive changes happening.

PHASE 4: Restoring control of your balance

In phase 4, we will now focus on helping you move for common day-to-day movements using the upper body for 25% of the workload, the mid back for 25%, the low back for 25% and the lower body for 25% (give or take).

We help you remind your muscles, spinal cord and subconscious mind of more energy-efficient ways to move that do not leave you out of breath, holding your breath or in pain.

PHASE 5: Restoring control of your body under higher loads

In the final phase we gradually expose your system to dynamic on-feet tasks and restore its ability to use many variations to achieve the same task giving it back movement options to achieve common tasks with increased load. We integrate the toe nail to finger nail and make sure you continue to integrate the concepts covered in phases one to four and earn the right to progress to phase 5. Phase 5 covers fundamental movements such as the squat and lunge since you perform some variation of those two movements every single day. We utilise more elastic energy and get everything doing its own job so your low back does not have to do all the work.

Now again, this may look like a very basic plan but 'genius demands simplicity'. I pride myself on doing the basics EXTRA-ordinarily and this is the problem for most complex cases I consult with. The patient has not earned the right to progress to the next level whereas the beauty of this system is that we build the foundation pillars first and foremost before moving onto movements that require these pillars to be in place. This ensures a natural progressive system that will allow you to achieve realistic changes and progress in both movement potential and pain levels.

CHAPTER 8

What can you expect from the 'Beat Back Pain and Sciatica without Pills, Injections or Surgery System'?

The patient's emotional graph is outlined below. This is the reality of the situation and is exactly why we require the mental preparedness from chapter 6.

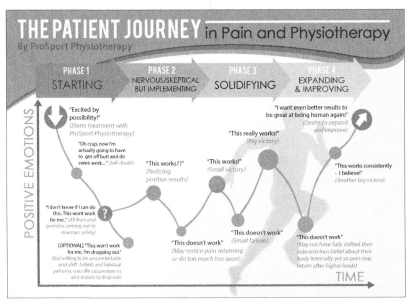

As you progress through this programme, you will have some small wins and some small setbacks. However, as you maintain your discipline, you will continue to gather even more momentum as you remind your body how it once was able to move with thoughtless, fearless movement.

You are excited at the moment at the possibility of this programme and the results that it can get for you. However, tomorrow morning when you wake up, the realisation may kick in that, actually, you need to do some work now in order to get to your own personal destination that motivates you. After a few days where there may or may not be noticeable changes in your symptoms and pain levels you begin to doubt yourself and this programme. 'I don't know if I can do this. This won't work for me' are common thoughts that might be running through your mind.

Then you might finally get a great night's sleep and have a small victory and your motivation and determination receives a boost again. This might be followed by a small increase in symptoms at a later point due to maybe increased activity and confidence. This can cause a small set-back again and the mindset may go back to self-doubt again.

However, right around the corner is a BIG victory that follows as you progress from stage to stage and you now see significant differences in your ability to move without fear, decreased pain levels and the ability to sleep better. But if you had succumbed to the doubt previously you would never have experienced this result; that, unfortunately, is the reality of the situation with the majority of patients on their road to restoring control of their body.

Remember if you listen to your heart you will succeed, but if you listen to your mind you will probably succumb!

If you perform this programme for at least 30 days, you will see some results. If you dedicate just 1% of your day (14 minutes) to the phase 2 work alone, you will give your body 15 minutes of mirroring a system that is in 'rest and digest'. The heart rate variability monitors I use to track when my patients have the highest stress reactions throughout the day can show me that people with persistent pain NEVER experience a 'rest and digest' dominance. However, when they simply following the phase 2 work their brain waves quieten and return to a gamma wave, and their heart rate variability and breathing variability increase. These are all signs that the system is predominantly in 'rest and digest'.

However, if we have the DISCIPLINE and motivation to implement phase 1 and control our thoughts and emotional reactions and use them as a trigger, we can actually instantly get into rest and digest and combine phases 1 and 2.

Will you be completely free of pain after 30 days?

It is too hard to say but I will guarantee you that if you perform these exercises and movements consistently then your system will adapt and will accept this 'rest and digest' dominance more readily and more consistently and you will restore the ability to move between both the 'rest and digest' and 'fight or flight' rather than letting one side dominate your life.

What about if my pain gets worse?

Your pain levels are affected by numerous factors and it is important to recognise this and reassure yourself that any one of the stressors to the system may impact the pain levels rather than just the tissues around the area of pain. Your range of motion around your back, your hips, your mid back and your shoulders may improve as you progress through the stages as the protective tone decreases. Therefore, as you challenge your movement capabilities it is common for the system to put down some new protective tone elsewhere in the body until it trusts you can control this new-found range of motion. It is important to acknowledge that this is part of the process of your journey to your destination. If there is a day where your pain levels are particularly high then revert back to your phase 1 and 2 exercises to ensure your system has NO OPTION but to get back to the 'rest and digest' dominance. If you have any doubt about your capabilities to perform the exercises then please get medical clearance prior to starting this programme.

When do I stop taking the pills?

This question is very much a conversation that needs to happen between you and your GP. You will however need to communicate your progress and desire not to be reliant on medications to your GP as they may be resistant to change anything at the moment. If they are resistant then their reasons for maintaining your medication need to be crystal clear and centered around your needs and not their stats or their needs.

What happens when I am pain-free?

That is a good problem to have! The accompanying website to the book will contain a special resource for patients who graduate from the 'Beat Back Pain and Sciatica without Pills, Injections or Surgery System' so we have you covered there and will help and guide you to move to your next programme, the Sustainability and Resilience Programme which we will be introducing you to in phase 5.

SECTION 3
Taking Action

CHAPTER 9

The breathing, moving, healing 5-phase approach to moving away from pain and towards a strong, resilient body and mind

PHASE 1: Restore control of your thoughts

Remember: Thoughts ⇨ Emotions ⇨ Behaviour. Therefore, we are now going to consciously break up this process at every opportunity we have and develop new habits so that instead of allowing your thoughts to bring your body into a state of 'fight or flight', we will now reframe your thoughts and bring new emotions and physiological reactions throughout your body.

In order to do this, we need to be very clear on where you want to get back to in life, how you want to feel and have a clear image in your mind of what this looks like.

Too many people 'don't want to be in pain' or 'don't want to feel this way'. But how do you actually want to feel? Remember this is like the analogy of setting the GPS to 'anywhere but London' when trying to get to Huddersfield. We need to set the GPS to the destination that you'd like to arrive at.

PHASE 1 Exercise 1: Establishing the destination

Write down below what your low back or painful area currently feels like but also what it feels like when you do day-to-day activities such as lifting, getting into bed or generally in everyday life (Hint: It might feel stiff, sore, wooden, like glass, rigid.)

1. _____

2. _____

3. _____

4. _____

5. _____

Write down below what your body as a whole currently feels like at present but also when you do day-to-day activities such as lifting or getting into bed or generally in everyday life (Hint: It might be wooden, heavy, stiff etc.)

1. _____

2. _____

3. _____

4. _____

5. _____

Finally write down below your most common moods and emotions that you currently feel on a day-to-day basis (Hint: You might feel angry, resentful, sad, tired or frightened.)

1. _____

2. _____

3. _____

4. _____

5. _____

Note: Please visit **www.breathingmovinghealing.com** and head to the resources section to download the audio file as I talk you through this next exercise. Or you may choose to read the section below a few times before closing your eyes and implementing it or, if you choose, ask a partner or friend to read out the following lines as you perform this exercise:

• Now I want you to close your eyes and recall a time in your life when your low back (or painful region) felt great, without pain and without any issues at all; this might be quite a few years ago, perhaps even when you were a child or teenager.

- As you recall this time, notice where you are.
- Notice who else is present.
- Notice the clothes you are wearing.
- Notice the weather on this particular day/evening.
- Notice if the image or movie is black and white or colour.
- Notice if the image or movie in your mind is close-up or far away.
- Now as you recall all these details and you focus on that image or movie, I want you to bring your attention to your low back or painful area.
- I want you to notice how it feels (remember the subconscious mind can't process negatives so don't say 'I don't have any pain' but rather describe how it feels with adjectives – for example, it might feel free, light, flexible, mobile etc.)
- Take a few more seconds and think about how your back feels and describe it in your own words below:

1. _____

2. _____

3. _____

4. _____

5. _____

- Good, you're doing great. Now think about your whole body and describe how it feels, again only using positives and in your own words:

1. _____

2. _____

3. _____

4. _____

5. _____

- Good, you're doing really well. Now think about your whole general mood and describe how it feels, again only using positives and in your own words:

1. _____

2. _____

3. _____

4. _____

5. _____

Now open your eyes and write down on the left-hand side of a blank page your first answers on what your back, whole body and mood feels like.

Then on the right-hand side of the page, write down how you want your lower back, whole body and mood to feel.

For most people, where they are now and how they feel is actually the complete opposite to how they want to feel or where they want to get to. For a lot of people in the clinic who do this exercise, they are surprised at how far back they had to go, and for some it can be emotional, so if you have tears right now, it's OK and you are not alone.

By performing the exercise above, you've already set the subconscious mind GPS coordinates to the destination you want to get back to, how you want your back to feel (even if you're a few years older now) and how you generally want to feel. Now let's start the engine and take the first mile of the journey with the next exercise.

PHASE 1 Exercise 2: Bringing the destination to the top of your mind little and often

The image or movie that came to your mind in the exercise above will now be used as a pattern interrupt to disrupt this vicious cycle of: pain ⇨ negative thoughts ⇨ negative emotions ⇨ negative behaviours.

We want to bring this powerful destination image or movie to the top of your conscious mind and hence also in your subconscious mind little and often (just like you'd constantly refer back to a GPS in your car throughout the journey).

Exercise 2a: Computer and phone background images

I would like you now to use either the destination image or a picture that easily reminds you of it as the background image on your phone screen and computer and anywhere else that you look at frequently throughout the day. If you spend a lot of time in one particular room, it might be worth printing off an image and getting it framed and placed on your mantelpiece or desk etc.

If you don't have a picture of the exact image that came up, you might consider googling the place you were at and using that picture, for example. The point is that the image is designed to instantly redirect your mind to the GPS or destination.

Exercise 2b: Phone and computer passwords

I would also like you to change your computer and phone passwords to meaningful numbers or phrases that again instantly redirect your mind to the destination you want to get back to.

Again this can seem a bit over the top but when the initial excitement of reading this book is finished, you need something there to constantly remind you (just like glancing at the GPS) to ensure you stay on the right track as you continue your journey.

PHASE 1 Exercise 3: Restore your thoughts to the destination

This exercise will be the most challenging exercise in phase 1; however, it will also be the most effective and fastest way to get you to the destination.

From this moment forward, every time you experience an unpleasant sensation or pain in your low back area or wherever your pain is located, I want you to become consciously aware of the thoughts that come into your mind. I then want you to become aware of the emotions and feelings those thoughts bring. If you are able to, I want you to write them down and be curious.

Now if you have a 'useless' thought or emotion, i.e. a negative thought or emotion that is not productive to getting you to the destination, I want you to overwrite this thought or emotion by bringing your attention to a 'useful' thought and hence emotion – that image or movie clip from exercise 1 above. You may even need to get your phone out and look at an image.

What this will do is break up the cycle of: pain ⇨ negative thought ⇨ negative emotion ⇨ negative or reinforced 'useless' behaviour and get you back to your destination.

From here on in, any time we experience that unpleasant sensation or pain experience, I want you to accept it for what it might be, a warning signal from your subconscious mind that your low back muscles and low back region are working very hard and want change, and that they may want other parts of your body to do their job so they don't have to continue to do excessive work.

So now we will get: pain ⇨ negative or 'useless' thought ⇨ negative or 'useless' emotion ⇨ awareness of these thoughts ⇨ positive or 'useful' thought ⇨ positive or 'useful' emotion ⇨ positive or useful behaviour (your body going back towards 'rest and digest').

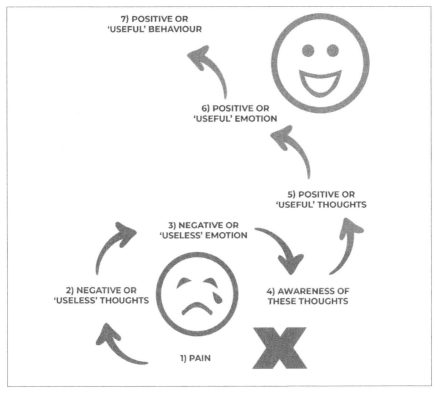

Now of course there will be times when you get pain and forget to restore your thoughts to the destination and the cycle of useless thoughts, useless emotions and useless behaviour continues but don't beat yourself up over that. That is in the past. The next time you have an unpleasant sensation or pain sensation, we will go again and disrupt this pattern with our powerful image or movie of the destination for your low back, body and mind.

I have learned the hard way that if we focus on phases 2–5 without first addressing phase 1 and clarifying exactly where we want to get to and regaining control of our thoughts, emotions and behaviour then this can be a very time-consuming process. If, however, we master phase 1 first, then the benefits of phases 2–5 can happen very quickly.

Now let's move even closer to our destination by progressing to phase 2 where we will integrate the powerful image or movie from phase 1 with some simple breathing exercises that can make a massive difference to our pain levels.

PHASE 2 Restore control of your respiratory system

Phase 2 is all about restoring mobility in your ribcage, mid spine, diaphragm and pelvic floor so these areas can contribute to your everyday movements so your low back doesn't have to do extra work.

For a lot of patients with back pain, bending forward to touch your toes or tie your shoe laces can be frightening and very painful in some instances. When we go to touch our toes, the same percentage analogy can be made here as before. Focusing on the spine and ribcage for now, when we bend forward the top of the spine would need to contribute 25% of the movement, give or take, the ribcage 25%, the mid spine 25% and the low back 25%. For a lot of people who are unable to relax the low back muscles, the low back would end up actually trying to do 75% of the work instead of its fair share. I believe this may then have the low back tissues communicating to your spinal cord and higher centres in your brain saying 'Hey, I'm doing most of the work here again; something needs to change' and ultimately you may have a pain sensation.

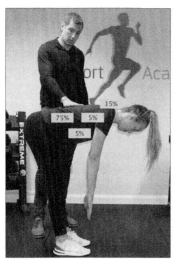

Here we see a person trying to touch their toes. The lower back muscles would want to lengthen here usually along with the abdominals, ribcage and neck flexors to help bring the person's fingers to their toes. Here we see the lower back muscles and neck muscles continuing to shorten, actually doing even more work than they need to do. This is a common way of moving for a lot of patients as they come into the clinic.

Now here's the interesting part...

One of the first tissues closest to your spine that has to lengthen when you go to bend forward is your diaphragm. When this lengthens, it allows your ribcage and mid spine to do 25% of the workload each. That's a massive 50% of the workload.

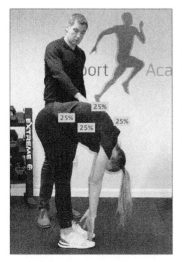

Now the ribcage and mid back can mobilise, the low back muscles are doing less work and the neck can also completely relax. The eyes and neck can orient towards the toes and help contribute to the momentum of the movement.

Here's the kicker, however. A lot of my patients who go to touch their toes anticipate pain and so they hold their breath before they move. Holding the breath actually does the complete opposite of what we want to happen at the diaphragm and actually shortens the diaphragm instead of allowing it to lengthen. This immediately impacts the ribcage and mid back's ability to contribute efficiently to the movement. Over time this action, combined with an increased breathing rate and an increased inhalation (volume of air that's been taken in) means that the diaphragm loses its ability to fully lengthen throughout the day or when you are sleeping. This may further impact the ribcage and mid spine and so the vicious cycle of the low back having to do extra work continues.

When you go to put your socks on at the edge of your bed in the morning, you need almost maximal mobility through the ribcage, hips and spine and so definitely need the diaphragm (and its partner the pelvic floor) to be able to go through a full range of motion. The good news is there are ways to help your diaphragm lengthen which I'll show you below but one of the best ways is to sit in a relaxed posture (that almost looks like you're slouching) throughout the day which we will also cover in the next phase. By stopping your thoughts from turning into negative emotions and going further into 'fight or flight', which naturally increases your breathing rate, then we also give the diaphragm and pelvic floor an opportunity to go through a full range of motion, along with the hip joints. The bottom line is if we can help mobilise these tissues, then we can help a lot of areas of the body do their jobs so the low back doesn't have to do excessive work, become grumpy and send excessive messages to your brain which contribute to you having a painful sensation.

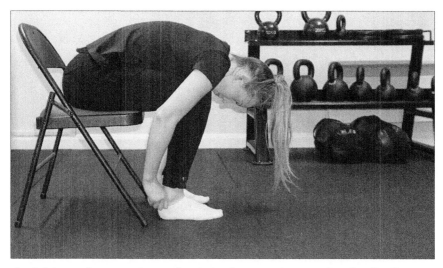

Activities such as putting socks on in the morning require the diaphragm to lengthen, the ribcage to mobilise and the low back muscles to relax. The more that this happens, the easier you should find it to do this movement without restriction or pain. The more you hold your breath when moving, the harder it is for the diaphragm to lengthen and the ribcage to mobilise.

Another big reason for wanting your ribcage and mid back along with your diaphragm to move through a full range of motion is that the more these move, the more the low back muscles will be able to relax and the lower body will be able to do more work as a whole. Now the lower body needs to work as a team and not just rely on one or two muscles to do the extra work which we will talk about later in phases 4 and 5.

OK, so let's get started and check your ability to lengthen your diaphragm with our first exercise which will require you to use a stopwatch on your watch or phone.

Phase 2 Exercise 1: Exhalation time trial

Sit on a chair in a reasonably comfortable position (if able) and get your stop watch ready to go.

Place your tongue on the roof of your mouth, lips together, teeth slightly apart (if you have no known obstructions in your nasal passages or know any other reason not to breathe through your nose) and take a normal breath in through your nose.

At the top of the breath and just as you are about to exhale, start the stopwatch and exhale through your mouth for as long as you can, stopping the stopwatch once you have finished exhaling. You can also do this test while exhaling through your nose and record the time which may be slightly longer.

Now record your time.

Exhalation time normal breath in through the nose, out through your mouth: _____

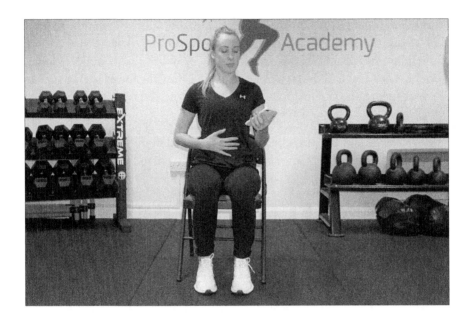

Record your exhalation time using the instructions above with a phone or stopwatch.

It is interesting to note that this is your conscious awareness of taking a full exhalation; said another way it is your ability to lengthen your diaphragm through a particular range of motion.

Now after a minute or so, once you have fully recovered, take another breath in and instead of exhaling through your mouth, this time I want you to keep your tongue on the roof of your mouth with your lips closed and make a prolonged humming sound while starting the stopwatch once you begin humming.

It's OK to smile while humming as it's perfectly normal to feel a bit silly doing this but smiling is good!

Now as you come to the natural end of the hum I want you to notice the time on the stopwatch but don't stop quite yet.

I want you to continue to hum and force every last little bit of air out of your body (your voice may even go a little bit croaky) and finally when all the air is well and truly out of your body, stop the stopwatch and record the time below, once you've had a chance to recover.

After this prolonged exhalation for the first time, it is natural for your breathing rate to increase slightly so as you inhale on the next breath, I want you to just focus on the air coming through the nostrils and slow the air as it comes in through the nose with the phrase 'I am safe' running through your mind. This will help slow your breathing rate down further.

Now, go ahead and record your time below.

Exhalation time normal breath in through the nose, and hum:

_____

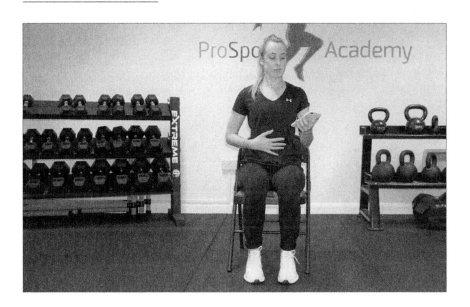

Record your exhalation time using the instructions above with a phone or stopwatch but this time hum either silently or out loud and notice the difference between the exhalation times.

It is not uncommon for a patient to treble, sometimes, quadruple their exhalation time with the help of a hum. This is because initially we are overriding your conscious mind in helping your diaphragm lengthen naturally by giving you a task of humming. Then when you get those feelings inside from your subconscious mind and body telling you that you are nearly at the end of the exhalation, you use your conscious mind to override your subconscious mind and force that last bit of air out that would never have got out otherwise.

So I hope you can see now that they are always playing off each other and the reality is we can actually lengthen our diaphragm a lot more than we consciously think which is why we need to be very particular with the types of stimulus we give our body rather than just basic 'sucking our belly button in' or 'switch your bum/glute muscles on' type exercises. If we give it the correct stimulus all of this stuff we happen naturally and you will get to move with thoughtless, fearless movement.

You can use our humming exercise above any time you want to get into 'rest and digest' and prolong your exhalation. Remember, inhalation is 'fight or flight' and exhalation is 'rest and digest'. We want to spend more time exhaling than inhaling. You can also do this exercise and hum silently if you are in a public place. The intention of humming silently is enough to get a similar effect. I tell a lot of my patients that any time they are stopped at a red light is a good opportunity to practice their humming and get further into 'rest and digest' while also lengthening the diaphragm.

Another great by-product of prolonged humming, which you may have felt towards the end of the hum, is that your tummy or 'core' muscles tighten and work. This is because these muscles' true function first and foremost is to help you breathe and keep you alive. Again we can subconsciously stimulate these muscles without needing to brace or activate them.

We will further strengthen these muscles in the next few exercises with the use of a balloon by again taking advantage of performing a task while getting our diaphragm to lengthen but also to add resistance to strengthen our abdominals in helping them to mobilise our ribcage, just like they need to be able to do when we bend over to pick something up or put our socks on.

For the next two exercises you require two balloons. Balloons come in various strengths depending on their quality but the stiffer, higher quality balloons with more resistance are the ones to look out for. Usually these will be the 10-pack of balloons sold at the same price as the 25-pack. There is nothing wrong with the 25-pack balloons but just be aware as you progress you will want the stiffer balloons to challenge you further so that you continue to progress towards your final destination.

Phase 2 Exercise 2: Balloon with hole exhalations

For the first exercise, I would like you to grab a pen or scissors or even use your fingernail and just prick a small hole in the balloon, at the furthest point away from the mouthpiece. It just needs to be a small nick so the balloon won't inflate completely but will inflate a small amount. Too big a hole and the exercise won't be as effective.

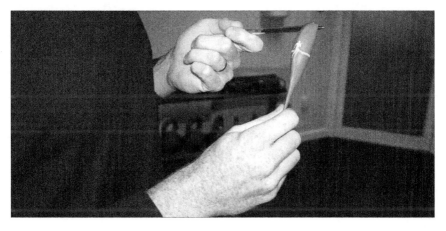

Prick a small hole at the end of the balloon either with a pen or something sharp.

Once ready you will lie on your back with your knees bent (if you are able to, or else sitting comfortably on a chair). Holding the balloon with your left hand, put it in your mouth and repeat the inhalation through the nose with the tongue on the roof of the mouth, lips together and teeth slightly apart.

Now blow into the balloon and continue to blow at a pace just fast enough to keep the balloon inflating the small amount as shown in the image below.

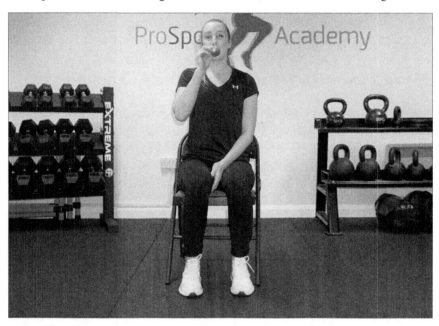

Exhale into the balloon and keep it inflating as if there was no hole in it. Maintain your exhalation for as long as possible keeping the balloon inflated to its maximum potential with the hole in it. This helps train the abdominal muscles subconsciously, while lengthening the diaphragm and mobilising the ribcage.

Once you've finished exhaling, keep the balloon in your mouth and pause for three seconds before lightly inhaling through the nose, focusing your attention on the air as it passes through the nostrils and slowing the air down as it passes through.

At the top of the inhalation, pause for a second and then repeat the exhalation through the balloon. Override the subconscious mind at the bottom of the exhalation and make sure all air is out of your lungs before pausing for three seconds at the bottom and slowing the air down through the nostrils through the inhalation again.

Repeat this exercise for a total of six full breaths before taking a short break of two to three minutes and repeating again twice more for a total of three sets.

You should notice that your exhalations are getting longer; you may even notice your ribcage is moving more freely as you exhale and that your tummy muscles (abdominals) are working.

Once you can do this exercise comfortably and control your inhalation then we will move to the next progression, this time without any hole in the balloon.

Phase 2 Exercise 3: Balloon exhalations

Once ready, lie on your back with your knees bent (if you are able to or else sitting comfortably on a chair). Holding the balloon with your left hand, put it in your mouth and repeat the inhalation through the nose with the tongue on the roof of the mouth, lips together and teeth slightly apart.

Now blow into the balloon and continue to blow at a pace just fast enough to keep the balloon inflating until your exhalation comes to a natural end. We want a slow, steady exhalation and the balloon inflating at a steady pace. The first breath might be tougher as you overcome the initial resistance of the balloon.

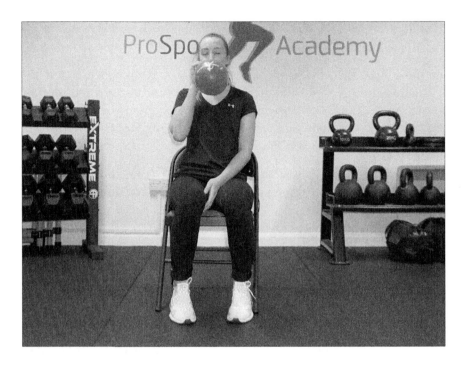

Now exhale into a balloon without any hole. Maintain a slow steady exhalation throughout, pausing at the bottom of the exhalation for three seconds before slowly inhaling again through your nose. This exercise provides even more resistance for the abdominals to work against whilst mobilising the diaphragm and ribcage.

Once you've finished exhaling, keep the balloon in your mouth and pause for three seconds before lightly inhaling through the nose, focusing your attention on the air as it passes through the nostrils and slowing the air down as it passes through.

At the top of the inhalation, pause for a second and then repeat the exhalation through the balloon. Override the subconscious mind at the bottom of the exhalation and make sure all air is out of your lungs before pausing for three seconds at the bottom and slowing the air down through the nostrils through the inhalation again.

Repeat this process until the balloon is fully inflated, ideally within two to three breaths. Now, this time, deflate the balloon to the side of your mouth (don't swallow the air) as you inhale through your nose with your lips closed, tongue on the roof of the mouth and your teeth slightly apart.

That is one repetition or one full balloon inflation. Repeat this process for a total of six full balloon inflations before taking a short break of two to three minutes and repeating again twice more for a total of three sets.

You should notice that your exhalations are getting longer; you may even notice your ribcage is continuing to move more freely as you exhale and that your tummy muscles (abdominals) are working really hard at the end of the exhalations.

SHORTCUT TO ARRIVE AT YOUR IDEAL DESTINATION QUICKER

For additional bonus points, and to get to your destination even quicker, at the end of your exhalations and as you slow the air as it comes in through your nostrils, ensure that your lower ribs don't rise forward towards the ceiling, if lying on your back, or your chest doesn't rise upwards, if seated on a chair. While continuing to inhale slowly and lightly, only inhale as much as you can keep the ribs and chest down. This may create a short air hunger feeling and may be a little unpleasant but will help strengthen the diaphragm further.

Don't worry too much about this initially as if you focus on slowing the air as it comes through the nostrils, then you will achieve a lot of this but as the exercise above becomes more comfortable, this is something I would encourage you to master.

Combining phases 1 and 2 for even faster results

Now we will combine restoring control of our thoughts along with restoring our most efficient breathing patterns to help you throughout the day but also to get you into 'rest and digest' before going to bed for a great night's sleep.

From my use of heart rate variability monitors with persistent pain patients, I could see that a lot of these patients were getting seven, eight or even nine hours sleep at times but still waking up feeling exhausted, stiff and lethargic because their autonomic nervous system was in 'fight or flight' throughout the night and actually expending energy and releasing cortisol (a stress hormone) rather than replenishing energy and healing their body and mind.

By helping you get into 'rest and digest' before you go to bed, then we can give you the best chance of shutting down the cortisol supply and replenishing your energy levels throughout the night so you actually wake up feeling energised, refreshed and more mobile.

This may take a few attempts before you are able to finally sleep through the night and wake feeling refreshed but a lot of my patients are amazed at the impact these simple drills can do.

The exercises below can also be used first thing in the morning if you have some 'brain fog' or are feeling exhausted, stiff and lethargic as a way to quieten the mind and oxygenate the body and all the muscles.

So with that said, let's get started.

Phase 2 Exercise 4: Attention check & trigger – to be completed throughout the day

The attention check and trigger exercise involves coming up with some form of trigger for you to bring your system into a state of 'rest and digest' frequently throughout your day. Think about it – more than likely your system has been in the habit of 'fight or flight' dominance for a certain period so any trigger that can break the HABIT and start a new one, bringing you into a state of 'rest and digest' is good. In this instance, we will use the triggers from phase 1 (images on your phone, password reminders etc.), but also any discomfort or pain as a trigger to check our attention and refocus.

Keeping your attention on useful thoughts can straight away help your pain. A good friend and top mind coach to numerous professional athletes,

Karl Morris, once said to me 'Your attention is either useful or useless.' We can help you change your story by keeping your mind on useful attention amongst other techniques below.

If we recall the GPS analogy and your subconscious brain directing you to the main destination, is the sum of all your thoughts and attention throughout the day 'useful' or 'useless' in getting you there? Now this isn't all about positive thinking as I completely appreciate it isn't as easy as this for someone living with persistent pain. But we can start to break the habits that have formed both on a conscious and subconscious level by using these triggers we'll talk about shortly to get you back into 'rest and digest'.

I hope you can now see that actually a quick fix magic exercise may not be out there but what is out there is a solution and hope. We need to understand that the human body works as one – if we only understand the muscles and joints of the body, we are well and truly missing the boat. This is why we have to influence the subconscious mind for long-lasting changes.

So for the attention, check and trigger exercise, I want you to write down the following question on a Post-it, whiteboard and various other places your eyes will glance at throughout the day.

Is my attention on 'useful' or 'useless' things that will help me get to my destination?

As you go through the day, you will become more aware of refocusing your thoughts and attention back to the image or movie of your ideal destination while doing 1–3 sets of humming.

Don't get frustrated, especially initially if you find your thoughts are indeed on things that are 'useless' in terms of getting you to your destination; this is normal and will change very quickly.

We will break this habit of having your attention on 'useless' thoughts while also getting your body further into rest and digest. We will mobilise the ribcage, diaphragm and pelvic floor and restore control of your mind and body with 'useful' thoughts which drive 'useful' emotions and cause you to take action with 'useful' behaviours.

Phase 2 Exercise 5: Bedtime and morning belief restoration – to be completed before going to bed and first thing in the morning before getting out of bed

Now most people struggle with meditation and the discipline required for meditation therefore I have adapted numerous approaches to mindfulness to come up with this five-step hybrid progression that is integrated into phase 2. It combines mindfulness with our unique breathing strategy in positions that will help restore the lengthening and shortening ability of the pelvic floor and diaphragm. When we allow the diaphragm to lengthen, the abdominals activate naturally which helps to relax the lower back muscle.

Now in addition to all these great things happening, what we are also doing is stimulating certain brain waves that are known to be more open to your suggestions and hence can access the subconscious mind even easier. If we recall that a big part of this low back pain sticking around for longer than it needs to is because the subconscious mind thinks there is still a threat present and refusing for the low back area to relax, then stimulating these brain waves and consciously communicating these belief statements to your subconscious mind may help speed this process up.

What you are actually doing here is a form of self-hypnosis. But don't worry. Hypnosis gets a bad rap due to the comic shows that have people on stage doing silly things. All you are doing is getting your body and mind in a relaxed state and attempting to communicate to your subconscious mind some simple beliefs that you want it to take on board in order to disrupt the thoughts ⇨ emotion ⇨ behaviour cycle. There is actually some really good evidence that hypnosis can help people with back pain but, as I said, it gets a bad rap due to the Hollywood movies. It is a form of relaxation and relaxation is something that we definitely want for you. Remember it is harder to relax than it is to tense.

So let's get started with your bedtime and morning routine.

[Please Note: there is a guided audio version of this and also a reference sheet to print out at **www.breathingmovinghealing.com** for your convenience.]

Step 1. Breathe lightly at all times through the nose, slowing the air as it travels through your nostrils with no greater than a 80% rate and depth of a 'conscious' normal breath. Slow it down and make the air even lighter as it passes through your nostrils.

Step 2. Keep your tongue on the roof of your mouth at all times slightly behind your teeth on the ridge of your pallet but not touching your teeth with your teeth slightly apart and lips gently pressed together no greater than 40% lip pressure.

Step 3. While focusing on a spot or something directly in front of you, instead of exhaling, hum for as long as possible for a total of three breaths until your ribcage is moving and you are beginning to feel relaxed. After three complete hums and when you are beginning to feel completely relaxed, revert back to breathing out through your nose and close your eyes, relaxing even further.

Step 4. Bring a loving memory or a memory of feeling safe into your heart and fill your body with that feeling (it may be the final destination image or movie, a memory of childhood, a pet, one of your children, your partner, whatever makes your heart tingle and makes you feel relaxed and happy). Breathe lightly and maintain discipline so your breathing is so light that you are unable to hear it and only inhale 80% of a maximum inhalation putting a cap on the inhalation so you have a small air hunger throughout your breathing.

Step 5. Repeat a belief that resonates with you with INTENT that engrains the new belief system you are trying to achieve (i.e. my body is becoming more and more mobile and fluid; my back is healing more and more every single day; my back is moving with even less pain every single day; I am strong and my body is resilient or, if you don't quite believe that yet, I am becoming stronger and stronger each day and my body is becoming more and more resilient each day).

Maintain the discipline of all four previous steps and recheck and reset if required as you repeat your belief statement ten times through.

By now your thoughts, emotions and body (behaviour) should be on 'useful' things, in 'rest and digest' setting you up for a great night's sleep or a great day ahead, getting you even closer to that ideal destination.

Reasoning behind the five-step belief system process

Step 1 ensures you are breathing lightly and therefore in a 'rest and digest' state with heart rate and diaphragm movement variability. Step 2 ensures that you maintain a nasal breathing pattern by keeping the tongue on the roof of the mouth which will also ensure the length-tension of all the muscles around your airway is optimal and allows you to swallow efficiently as required when performing this process. Breathing and swallowing processes are closely interrelated in their central control and are highly coordinated with many muscles and structures having dual roles, therefore it is vital we keep the correct tongue position for swallowing throughout our breathing work. In step 3 we further ensure you are in 'rest and digest'; by getting your eyes involved, we are stimulating the majority of your cranial nerves in your brain to synchronise and work together. In step 4, we intensify the feelings of safety and love to further bring your body into a state of 'rest and digest' and further away from 'fight and fight' so your whole body feels safe and your subconscious mind knows this before hearing these suggestions and belief statements. We maintain a slight air hunger by not fully inhaling and maintaining this breathing depth lightly to decrease the sensitivity of the respiratory messengers and allow them to get used to inhaling less air and making full use of the inhaled air. Step 5 reinforces these new beliefs with intent while your system is in a relaxed 'non-threatening' state and your brain waves have dropped to alpha and theta waves and are more open to learning new beliefs/suggestions with the use of the imagery from your destination image or movie.

Please visit **www.breathingmovinghealing.com** where I have recorded an audio version of this exercise for you to follow along to and download to use at a convenient time for you. Listening on headphones and following along can be very useful to keep your attention on the important points to get the most out of this exercise.

Each step above ensures you do the basics EXTRA-ordinarily without relying on fancy tricks and you earn the right to progress to the next phase of the programme. This five-step process should also be used during any times where your pain levels are high or particularly uncomfortable. This is a great time to get your system out of 'fight or flight' and back to 'rest and digest' and repeat a belief statement such as 'all parts of my body is safe' or 'all parts of my body reflect the feeling of a relaxed safe human being' to take your subconscious mind to a different place from being in 'perceived threat'.

I would like to acknowledge the work of Lois Laynee, Chris Walton, Grace Smith and Konstantin Buteyko for introducing me to their approaches, which I have then gone on to adapt and integrate to formulate my own belief restoration protocol above that I use on a daily basis with patients.

Updating the belief system might seem like the 'whackiest' or 'strangest' part of this whole system and for a lot of people this might be outside their comfort zone. But in reality, it is my opinion, even with sports people, that what we are really doing, even with a straightforward ankle sprain and its rehabilitation exercise plan, is showing the person's brain that the tissues are healing and it's safe to use them again. Essentially updating their belief system reduces the amount of swelling the body produces, allows the muscles to fire and coordinate in an optimal manner with the rest of the body and enables the person to consciously grow in confidence as a result.

There is no right or wrong time or place to perform this belief system restoration protocol – you can perform it anytime and anywhere. I recommend doing it at times when you want to reduce your pain and before going to bed to take your system to a place of 'rest and digest'.

PHASE 3: Restoring a relaxed low back while sitting and standing

So now we have taken care of the two biggest and most overlooked components to getting someone back to feeling strong and resilient – their thoughts/beliefs and their autonomic nervous system, we can now earn the right to progress to getting the rest of the body to move in a more efficient manner without trying to fight the subconscious mind and autonomic nervous system.

In phase 3 we are going after the big elephants in the room and getting the ribcage, mid spine and upper spine to do their jobs while sitting or standing and take some of that workload off the lower back.

I have learned the hard way that skipping this step and going straight to phase 4, while continuing with the activities that we do 10+ hours a day, is of very limited value. If we work hard throughout the day on phases 1 and 2 and then also implement phase 3, then these three phases alone can have a massive impact on people's lives.

Then phases 4 and 5 are the final pieces of the puzzle. Start with phase 4 without implementing phase 1, 2 and 3 and it's like trying to run uphill into a gale-force wind. OK, hopefully you get the idea and message by now – don't skip steps because they are all important.

So let's get started and get you even closer to your ideal destination.

Relaxed sitting

This may seem strange that we are looking at your sitting posture first and I can almost guarantee this next exercise is not what you think. In fact it will probably be the complete opposite to what you think is the 'right way to sit'. I might even upset a few therapists with these next exercises but hopefully you will try these with an open mind and feel the benefits immediately.

To get straight to the point, there is no 'perfect posture' or correct way to sit. An ideal posture is a posture that is always changing and an ideal way to sit is in a relaxed manner that allows you to be and feel comfortable.

Now what do the majority of people do instead? They sit up straight like they were told to do in school or by their parents. Last night at the dinner table, my wife Georgina, even told my daughter Ava to 'sit up straight and eat your dinner' to which she responded and sat bolt upright!

Now what's the problem with sitting bolt upright?

Do me a favour – if you are able to, sit bolt upright and even exaggerate this tall, upright stiff posture.

Now feel the muscles that run parallel to either side of your spine. You should notice that these muscles feel tense and are working hard to maintain this posture for you.

Now this is where we go back to the analogy of squeezing your fist for a period of time. After a while, maybe a few minutes even, these muscles are going to give you a conscious feeling or sensation and you are going to want to relax your fist and these muscles, right?

Well, the same thing happens with the low back muscles. They will give your spinal cord and brain signals/messages to say, 'Hey any chance I can relax for a few minutes and take a break?' or something along those lines. This may present in the form of an unpleasant sensation around your lower back and legs or even a painful sensation.

Now I also want you to reflect and look at this stiff, upright, tense posture and ask yourself if this is how you want your body to feel at your ideal destination from phase 1. For the majority of people, they are continuing to reinforce their reality with how their back feels today with how they sit and stand.

For most people, they want their low back area to feel relaxed, mobile, springy and free and yet are spending 10+ hours a day in stiff, tense, upright positions due to false beliefs that slouching is bad for us and our backs. In the medical world, there is actually no proof that I'm currently aware of that a slouched posture causes pain.

93

Now think of a person who is slouched and describe how they look and how you'd imagine them to feel? Words like relaxed and chilled out come to my mind. What about yours? Are these words that come to your mind getting closer to your ideal destination?

Now don't get me wrong, we don't want you to get into an extremely slouched posture that's completely the other way but we certainly want to find a happy medium that allows your low back muscles to actually relax when you're sitting (fist open and not tensed constantly) and your other body parts also relaxed so it's not actually costing you excessive energy to sit for 10+ hours a day.

So before we help you restore a relaxed sitting posture I want to highlight two of the most common and unproductive or 'useless' sitting postures I see that won't help you get to your destination anytime soon.

1 Sitting bolt upright with the two low back muscles running parallel along your spine fully active and tense as we covered above (think closed tight fist).

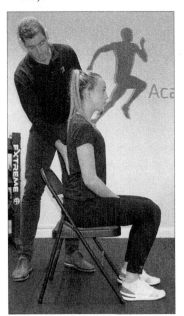

As you sit bolt upright, notice how this posture makes you want to almost hold your breath. Now feel the muscles either side of your spine as they run up towards your mid back. These muscles need to work hard to keep you in this posture. Think of these like clenching your fist for a prolonged period. After a while, just like the muscles holding your fist tightly clenched, they will start to fatigue and you may even get an unpleasant sensation coming from that area shortly after.

2 Sitting in the chair and it looks like your back is relaxed but you are actually pushing your back into the back of the chair. This again is activating your low back muscles (think closed tight fist again) as these muscles are constantly working. In this instance I like to joke with patients that they are supporting the chair rather than the chair is supporting them. With this posture, you again should be able to feel the muscles running up your low back quite active while sitting.

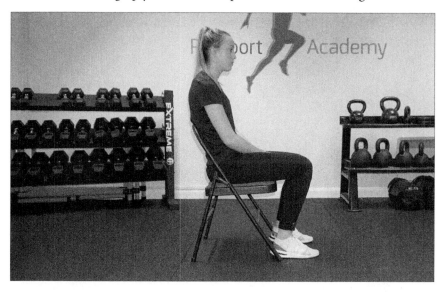

In this posture, although it looks like you are relaxed the low back pushing back into the chair is doing the same job as the clenched fist again and is having to work very hard, even though the chair is actually supposed to be supporting you.

Now let's retrain your body and mind how to relax these low back muscles, unclench the fist so to speak, and allow your body to be supported by the chair rather than you supporting the chair.

Phase 3 Exercise 1: Back tensing and relaxing while sitting

Sit bolt upright in a chair with your feet firmly planted on the floor.

Now place one hand on the lower back muscles that run along close to your spine and the other hand on your chest bone.

Notice how active the low back muscles are.

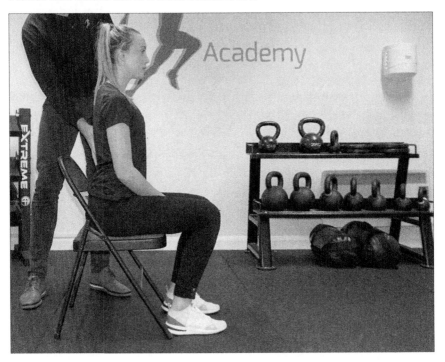

Notice how the low back muscles are behaving as you sit up straight.

Now take a nice slow inhale through your nose and as you exhale through your nose or mouth very gently guide your chest bone down to the floor if your pain sensation allows.

Notice how your low back muscles react and you should notice that these muscles actually begin to relax (or in other words, the fist relaxes and loosens its grip).

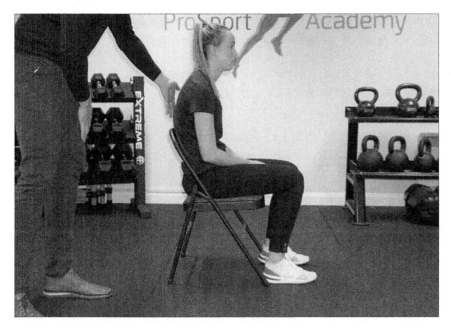

Notice as you exhale and the chest bone drops gently that the low back muscles actually start to relax.

Now gently guide your chest bone with your hand again up towards the ceiling or back to the start position and notice how your low back muscles react again.

Notice how these muscles will work again (or in other words, the fist tightens again).

Repeat this process of guiding your chest bone down and up, just a few inches and noticing the tensing and relaxing of your low back muscles to each movement.

Isn't it funny, don't you think, that when your lower back muscles are actually in the most relaxed state, this is also the posture that we have been told for decades is bad, when in actual fact it is a posture that allows our body and mind to completely relax.

This is also the posture that allows your diaphragm to stretch, your ribcage and mid spine to mobilise and contribute to the sitting posture instead of your lower back doing all the work. Hopefully by now you are beginning to see why we did phase 2 working on mobilising your ribcage and diaphragm before doing this exercise.

If you had an unpleasant sensation such as pain in your lower back region when guiding your chest bone to the floor, your diaphragm, ribcage and mid spine may need more help in mobilising and more work in phase 2 would be indicated along with progressing to the exercise below.

So now we need to find a happy medium which allows you to sit in a posture that feels comfortable and allows your low back muscles to actually relax throughout the day without feeling as if you're a stroppy teenager sitting with attitude!

Phase 3 Exercise 2: Back relaxed while sitting

So this exercise will do exactly what it says on the tin, allow your lower back to relax while sitting.

Now I want you to sit back into your chair so the base of the spine is right back into the chair and your feet are ideally planted on the floor.

Now take a slow, light inhalation through your nose and pause at the top of the inhalation for a second.

Now instead of exhaling I want you to instead let out a long 'sigh' or prolonged 'ahhhhh' as the air releases from your mouth. As you do so, I want you to let your whole body relax and let your shoulders drop as you make the sound.

Now hold that position and repeat a slow light inhalation and hold at the top for a second or two.

Now repeat the 'sigh' or 'ahhhhh' again and further relax your shoulders and body.

Now hold that position and repeat a final slow, light inhalation and hold at the top.

Now for the final time, repeat the 'sigh' or 'ahhhhh' and let your body completely relax and shoulders drop if they feel like they want to.

What you should notice is that you are in a more slouched position than when you started and your chest bone has dropped naturally towards the floor subconsciously, your diaphragm is in a more lengthened position, your ribcage has dropped and your mid spine has also contributed to the seated posture.

As you sit in this position, it is completely normal for it to feel completely alien to you and just plain 'wrong'.

But as you continue to sit here and your body gets used to it, notice how much more relaxed you feel.

Notice how your breathing rate is naturally starting to slow down.

Notice how your low back muscles have started to relax more.

Notice how your mid back, ribcage and abdominals are doing more of the work in this posture.

There are a whole lot of benefits to this exercise and I also want to bring to your attention how much work it takes to completely relax. Some people might need five to six 'sighs' or 'ahhhs' if they have had a particularly stressful day. Now that you are in a more relaxed posture, your breathing rate is slowing down and your body is beginning to relax and reenergise you so you can watch television, drive your car or do whatever it is you are doing while in a seated position.

Now for most people when you get into your car, or sit down to watch television or to eat your dinner, you may need to spend 60 seconds repeating this exercise to remind your body to relax initially. You may even need to adjust the car mirrors with your new relaxed posture. Then as your body gets used to this new relaxed posture, it will begin to feel less 'alien' and more normal which should also coincide with less unpleasant sensations around your lower back area.

It will take a little commitment but the more you sit in a relaxed posture with your low back relaxed and all the other parts of the body contributing to the movement, the more you are reinforcing 'useful' behaviour that is getting you closer to your ideal destination.

Sitting and standing

Now that you are sitting in more 'useful' positions throughout the day, we want to also further reinforce good movements where we not only get the ribcage, mid and upper back involved but also the lower body.

So what we are going to do now is allow your low back to continue to stay relaxed and ensure that your lower body does the majority of the work when standing. I will give you a couple of cues to imagine when standing to ensure that all the muscles in your lower body contribute to the movement and you don't put excessive pressure on your knees which I see a lot of patients do when they first come to our clinic.

Before we do that I want to show you a couple of ways that are not useful to stand to help you get to your destination.

A lot of patients when they go to stand up put the majority of pressure through their heels. As they stand up then, their knees usually come back to their heels and then the low back muscles have to react to keep them balanced and straighten them up. From my observations, this way of standing also uses your quad muscles a lot more than the rest of the muscles in your lower body and can tend to make some patients' knees sore.

A small number of patients will do the complete opposite and actually lift their heels off the ground and push with their toes to stand. This again will use the quad muscles excessively and, from my experience, will over time irritate the knees of some patients, but not all.

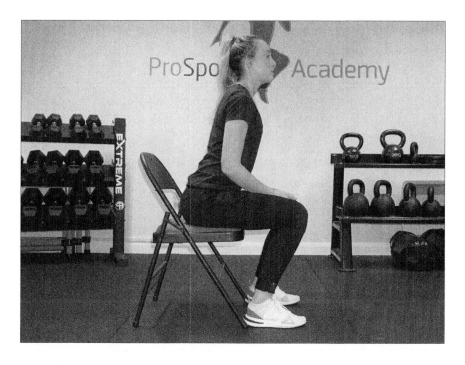

A lot of patients with back pain will hold their breath just as they are about to move. This contributes to the mid back going rigid and tightening the lower back. They then either push through the heels or excessively through the toes which further causes the lower back muscles to have to do more work as the patient stands each and every day.

So just like everything else that we are doing, we simply want everything to do its own job, nothing more, nothing less, while allowing the low back muscles to relax.

So now, before we proceed to the next exercise, stand up and notice how you usually stand up and also notice if your low back muscles are tensed or relaxed?

OK, so now let's get started getting everything else to do their jobs so the low back doesn't need to do too much work.

Phase 3 Exercise 3: Sitting and standing with a relaxed back

Sitting comfortably in a chair (the new relaxed way), I want you to slightly shuffle forward on the chair if need be to ensure that your midfoot is directly under your knee (midfoot is where the laces on your shoes are). Your knees may even be slightly over your toes now. That's fine.

Now I want you to tuck your chin to your chest and keep it tucked throughout the next few steps. This will further allow your lower back to relax and avoid it cheating and trying to get involved as you go to stand up.

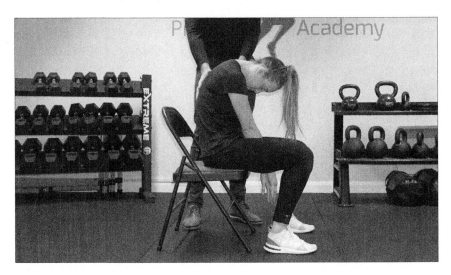

Start on the edge of the chair with your chin tucked, naturally allowing your shoulders and mid back to follow. Keep your weight and intent over your midfoot.

Now as you go to stand up, I want you to imagine you are squashing an orange under each midfoot where the laces are in your shoes. As you squash the orange into the floor, you should feel your bum muscles engage and your bottom rising from the chair.

Continue to squash the oranges with your midfoot, ensuring that you are not putting any pressure through your heels of your feet although they are still planted on the floor throughout the movement.

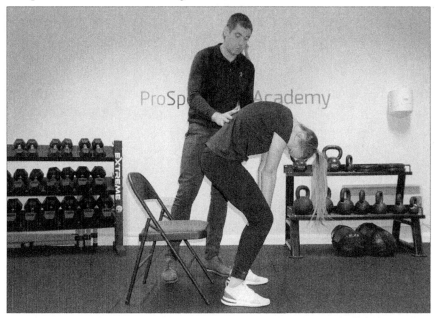

Continue to imagine squashing an orange through the midfoot while keeping the chin tucked and the mid back relaxed as you continue to rise up from the chair.

As you continue to squash the oranges, keep your chin tucked and your back relaxed throughout the movement so that as you stand upright, your chin is still tucked, your chest bone is still down slightly towards the floor and your low back muscles are still relaxed.

At the top of the movement you should almost feel like you have to do a small reverse curl and gently lift your chest bone up towards the ceiling slightly, to fully straighten if you completely relax your back throughout the movement.

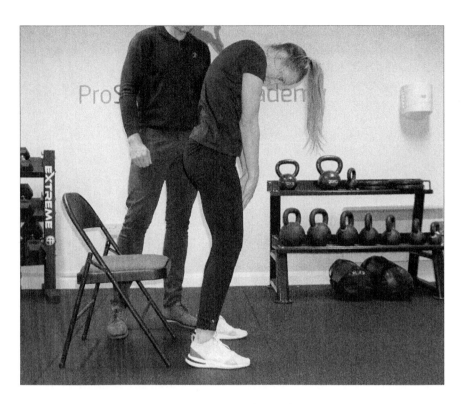

At the top of the movement, continue to keep the chin relaxed until the last second. You should notice all your weight is on your midfoot and you are doing a reverse curl of your neck to finally straighten up. This allows your lower back muscles to do as little as possible during the movement and gives the other muscles no option but to do their fair share of movement. Patients usually notice, the more work other body parts do, the less pain sensations they experience.

If you require the assistance of something like a table to help you up that's fine but I still want you to really focus on the steps above while using the aid to a minimum so your lower body muscles do most of the work.

For a lot of people, getting each part of the body to do its job and switching to this way of moving can have a massive impact on their pain sensations when standing up or getting out of a car. In the car scenario, your legs would not be completely side by side but the same principles apply; squash an orange through the midfoot and keep the chin tucked and use the door or whatever else as needed but have good intent through your midfoot while the chin remains tucked under.

On the way back down, all you need to do is reverse engineer the process. We start with the weight through the midfoot and as you go to sit down, tuck your chin to your chest and allow your chest bone to naturally drop towards the floor.

Now the only thing we do differently on the way down is we allow your weight to transfer back towards the heels while gently pushing your knees forwards over your toes to maintain balance as you descend down to the chair. Please ensure that as you are about to sit down, the weight distribution is roughly 60% on your heels and 40% on your midfoot where your laces are, down to your toes.

I have put a demo of this exercise inside your resource book which is available to download at **www.breathingmovinghealing.com**

Phase 3 Exercise 4: Standing with equal weight distribution between legs

The final exercise in phase 3 is a short one but very important for people who are standing for large periods of the day.

As you are now standing, if you feel confident to do so and your balance allows, close your eyes and feel how much pressure is on your left and right midfoot.

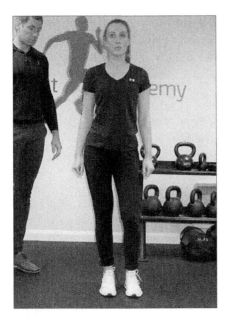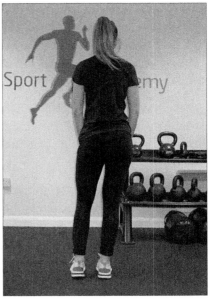

Notice how the majority of the body weight is being supported on the right heel. The left leg is contributing very little to this standing posture. Although this is OK short-term, for someone with lower back pain, we want to restore the ability of everything to do its own job to avoid any areas having to do excessive work while the pain sensation settles down.

Now gently adjust the pressure so that 50% of your body weight is being supported by your left midfoot and 50% by your right midfoot. Once balanced, quickly check your chest bone position and gently guide it down slightly to further relax the low back muscles. You should notice that your lower body will relax and take more of your body weight now.

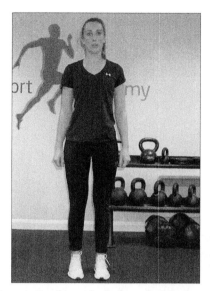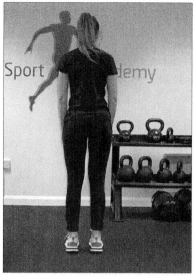

Now notice how the left and right legs are both contributing to the load management and avoiding any one area doing excessive work while the pain sensation is still present.

You may need to check in on this exercise throughout the day as, if you have had previous injuries to any muscles or joints in your lower limb, then it is common for your brain to try to protect these areas still and avoid using them. The problem is, another part of the body needs to compensate and the low back muscles are usually what take up the slack.

So, there you have it and congratulations for completing phase 3. As I mentioned, if you apply these exercises in phase 3 daily, combined with phases 1 and 2, there can be some remarkable changes in your pain sensations and how your body is beginning to move. This will set us up nicely for phase 4 which is where we start to get a little bit more specific to your story and your actual needs.

But remember, master and implement phases 1–3 before proceeding to phase 4 or you may get stuck in a traffic jam on the way to your ideal destination.

PHASE 4: Restoring control of your balance

So now that you are moving in the right direction of your ideal destination for 10+ hours a day sitting down and getting up and down from chairs, it's now time to show your brain that it's safe to load all the muscles in your lower body again.

You see, when we have an injury or pain in a body part, what we think happens is that the brain tries to protect this region (think limping after rolling your ankle) and decides not use certain muscle fibres around the injured area, or those above or below, that might put stress or load on the injured area.

What's really interesting, and also really important for you to get to your ideal destination, is that research has shown that once the pain or injury goes, some of these muscle fibres are still in protection mode, as if the injury is still present. Now that might be OK short term, but longer term what are the consequences? Well, for starters, other parts of the muscle may have to work harder and joints above and below may also have to compensate. So what we need to do is show your subconscious mind and spinal cord that it's safe to use these muscle fibres again. Now don't worry if you can't remember all your injuries in the past, for now. That won't become important until phase 5 as in phase 4 we are going to put your body into specific positions and force all your muscles to react in the different ways they will need to in real life.

Remember, although by now you may be noticing some dramatic improvements in your pain sensations and confidence as you move better, all we are really doing is reminding your subconscious mind and body how it is supposed to operate in order for you to live a pain-free and resilient life. We are simply giving it back what it once had, that's all and it's the exact same approach in phase 4.

Now before we do these movements, there are some simple rules which you must follow initially in order to get the most from them:

Rules of weight shift distribution:

- Slow the speed down so you can feel every inch of the foot working through the movements

- Keep looking at a spot on the wall in front of you and trust your body

- Find the contact point while breathing lightly throughout the whole movement

- Feel the sensation of your tissues in the hips and stomach throughout the whole movement

- Tongue on the roof of the mouth, lips together and breathing through the nose throughout the whole movement

- If you are apprehensive and worried about your balance, feel free to initially do these exercises near a table or wall to grab hold of if the need arises.

Phase 4 Exercise 1: Forward and back weight shift foot pressures

Start with your feet shoulder width apart and your hands by your sides. Rearrange your body weight so that your body weight is 50% on your left foot and 50% on your right foot and all the pressure is along the midfoot where the laces on your shoes would be.

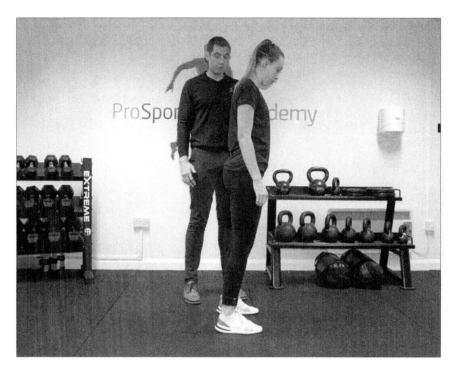

Start with your weight 50% on each leg and the pressure through the midfoot/laces region. As you adjust you may notice your weight come off your heels and your body travel forward slightly.

Exhale for as long as you can and towards the end of the exhalation slowly allow your whole body weight to travel forwards from your midfoot to the toes without the heels coming off the floor or breaking at the waist. Do this super slow so you can feel every inch of the movement with your feet.

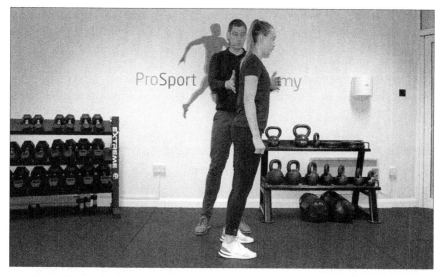

As you exhale, allow your weight to shift forward to the front of your foot without your heels lifting off the ground.

Now at the end of the movement, gently push with your toes and midfoot again and slowly allow your body weight to transfer towards the heels without your toes coming off the floor as you inhale through the movement.

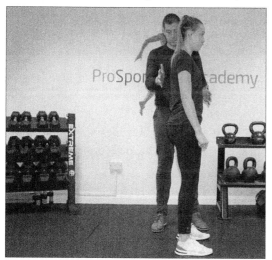

As you inhale, allow your weight to slowly pass through the midfoot towards the heels without your toes lifting off the ground.

At the end of the movement, when the majority of your weight is on your heels without your toes coming off, exhale and allow your body weight to travel from the heels super slow all the way forwards towards the toes as you exhale.

Repeat this back and forth movement for ten nasal breaths so five times forwards and back.

Phase 4 Exercise 2: Forward weight shift foot pressures with reach overhead

Now that you have felt the complete foot working and managing your body weight, it's time to get the upper body involved to challenge your base of support and balance further.

Start in the start position as previously. This time instead of moving your whole body as one, reach both hands up to the ceiling so you feel a gentle stretch in your tummy/stomach muscles. Please note if you are feeling pain in the lower back it is because you are probably not reaching up enough and too far back. As you reach up, inhale lightly and slowly for as long as possible through your nose synchronising the reach with the breath.

Now, as you reach up and can't reach up any more, then, and only then, start to reach your hands behind you overhead.

As your hands begin to reach upwards and your tummy starts to stretch, you should notice your weight shifts forwards slowly towards your toes again. As you bring your hands down, the weight should shift back to the midfoot again.

Slow the reach upwards so you have a greater awareness of the pressure changing in your feet and can feel as much of the tummy muscles stretch as possible.

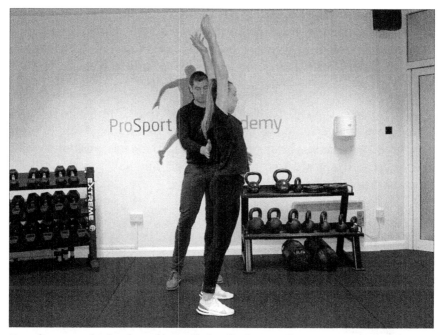

Reach upwards slowly, taking all the slack out of your tummy muscles until you feel a gently stretch around your stomach as your weight shifts forwards towards your toes without your heels lifting off the ground.

If you are unable to do this movement still due to the pinch in your lower back then you may need some help mobilising your ribcage further and focus more on phase 2, especially with the balloon exercises but also please reach out to us in the breathing, moving, healing support group inside your free member's area at **www.breathingmovinghealing.com**.

Phase 4 Exercise 3: Posterior weight shift foot pressures with reach forwards

Now it's time to get the upper body challenging your base of support and to balance further when you reach forward.

Start in the start position as previously. This time instead of moving your whole body as one, reach both hands forwards in front of you so you feel a gentle movement of your hips in the opposite direction and perhaps a gentle stretch in your hamstring muscles at the back of your thighs. As you reach forward, exhale lightly and slowly for as long as possible through your nose synchronising the reach with the breath.

As your hands begin to reach forwards and your hamstrings starts to stretch, you should notice your weight shifts backwards slowly towards your heels again. As you bring your hands back to the start position by your sides, squash an orange with your midfoot to get your hips to travel forwards again, bringing you back to the start position.

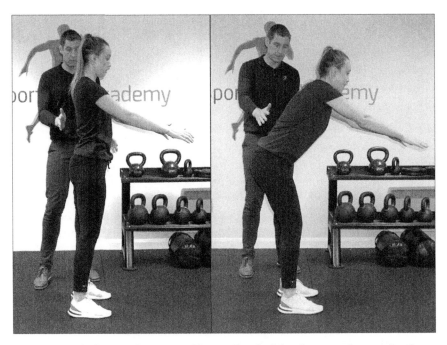

As you reach forwards, notice the weight shift back towards your heels. Ensure your toes do not come off the ground during the movement.

Slow the reach forwards again so you have greater awareness of the pressure changing in your feet and can feel as much of the hamstring muscles stretch as possible while exhaling throughout.

If you are unable to do this movement still due to the pinch or pain in your lower back then you may need some help mobilising your ribcage further by focusing more on phase 2, especially with the balloon exercises but also please reach out to us in the breathing, moving, healing support group inside your free member's area at **www.breathingmovinghealing.com**.

Phase 4 Exercise 4: Sideways weight shift foot pressures with reach down

Now it's time to get the upper body challenging your base of support and balance further in a side to side direction.

Start in the start position as previously with the weight evenly distributed 50/50 and all the weight on each midfoot.

This time reach your left hand down the outside of your left knee so you feel a gentle movement of your hips in the opposite direction and perhaps a gentle stretch on the outside of your right hip or even abdominal muscles by your ribcage. As you reach down, exhale lightly and slowly for as long as possible through your nose synchronising the reach with the breath.

As your hand begins to reach down, you should notice the weight goes more towards the inside of the left foot and the outside of the right foot.

There should also be a reaction where the hips move towards and eventually finish over and slightly outside the right foot.

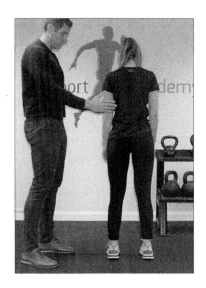 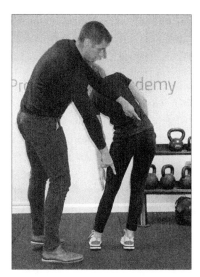

Notice as you reach your left hand down your left leg, your right hip should react and move outside your right foot without either foot losing contact with the floor.

As you bring your hands back to the start position by your sides, squash an orange with your right midfoot to get your hips to travel left again and bring you back to the start position.

If you notice that your hips don't travel to the right, then instead of reaching your left hand down, place it instead on your left outside lower ribs and gently push your whole body to the right so that your hips follow and you feel a stretch on the right outside abdominal region or right outside hips. You may need to do this a few times before rechecking the left hand reach by your side and you may notice that this time your hips move to the right as your left hand reaches down outside your left leg.

If you are unable to do this movement still or you are limited due to a pinch or pain in your lower back then you may need some help mobilising your ribcage further by focusing more on phase 2, especially with the balloon exercises but also please reach out to us in the breathing, moving, healing support group inside your free member's area at **wwwbreathingmovinghealing. com** where we will be able to direct you to some specially trained therapists who can speed this process up for you.

Repeat the same movements above with the right side, reaching your right hand down your right side and observing the reactions that happen in the rest of the body.

Phase 4 Exercise 5: Turning weight shift foot pressures

Now it's time to get the upper body challenging your base of support and balance further in a turning or twisting direction.

Start in the start position as previously with the weight evenly distributed 50/50 and all the weight on each midfoot. This time look over your right shoulder with your neck and allow your whole body to turn as if looking over your right shoulder very slowly.

Exhale gently through your nose slowly as you turn your body to the right; notice your left foot pressure changes towards your left big toe and your right foot pressure changes from the midfoot to now moving towards your right outside heel. You should also notice that your left knee might start to twist inwards gently and your right shin and thigh muscles may start to twist outwards.

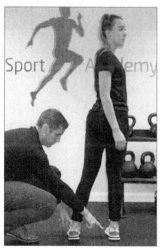

As you twist and look over your right shoulder, does the weight transfer over to your right heel without your right big toe losing contact with the ground? As you twist to the right, do you also feel the weight going towards your left big toe? These are some common reactions that happen with a lot of people during these movements to help to distribute the load efficiently.

As you come back to the start position, notice how the weight shifts from the outside right heel back towards the midfoot and the left foot pressure shifts from the big toe towards the midfoot.

If you notice that your knee or shin or thigh bones aren't moving gently or that you are not getting any pressure onto your right outside heel, then feel free to help your ribcage twist a little more gently with your hands. You may need to do this a few times before rechecking the movement without needing to help the ribcage move and you should now hopefully notice the reactions happening as described above with your bones and feet.

If you are unable to do this movement still or you are limited due to a pinch or pain in your lower back then you may need some help mobilising your ribcage further by focusing more on phase 2, especially with the balloon exercises but also please reach out to us in the breathing, moving, healing support group inside your free member's area at **www. breathingmovinghealing.com** where we will be able to direct you to some specially trained therapists who can speed this process up for you.

Repeat the same movements above twisting to the left side this time and observing the reactions that happen in the rest of the body.

These five exercises can be done two to three times a day and are great to do straight after your morning belief restoration protocol. Some of the variations can also be done throughout the day if you need to stand for prolonged periods to shift your weight around and wake up all the various muscles.

Ideally to progress to phase 5, we would want all the reactions that we described above to be happening and if you were in my clinic or working with any of the therapists specially trained by me then this would be the main focus before progressing onto phase 5 where we start to increase the load on these particular tissues.

If you are still unable to load these various tissues and get these various reactions as mentioned above, don't worry; it may just be that your subconscious mind is still protecting some of these tissues or that your ribcage is not mobile enough yet.

What these movements should highlight to you is how everything from the fingernail to the toenail is connected and how there are numerous reactions that have to happen throughout the body during day-to-day life. It should also highlight the importance of ribcage mobility and how, when we help this move, the rest of the body will change instantly, especially how much less work the lower back will do as a result.

If you stagnate at this phase then do please login to the support group on Facebook and let us know and we will be able to help you further specific to your needs.

Once you have practised these movements and the reactions mentioned above are happening, what this tells us is that your brain and subconscious mind are happy for your body to challenge their base of support and that you have increased your movement variability. This will again continue to decrease excessive workload on certain tissues and accelerate you closer to your ideal destination.

Remember to stick to the rules of the weight distribution at the start of this chapter and keep everything slow so you have greater awareness of the reactions of your feet and the rest of your body.

PHASE 5: Restoring control of your body under higher loads

Now we progress to phase 5 and we start to increase the speed of the movements and expose you to more functional movements that daily life requires. As always, the same rules apply – we want to ensure that all the muscles are doing their own jobs, nothing more, nothing less, and that your respiratory system (breathing patterns) communicates and works well with your muscles and joints.

As I mentioned at the end of the last chapter, I don't like personally to start this phase until the patient has passed the reactions mentioned in phase 4; however, even if you still aren't noticing all the reactions happening, I believe this phase can still help you reduce pain and encourage more energy-efficient movements.

The rules for phase 5 are below.

Phase 5 Rules:

- Always breathe during the movement
- Breathe lightly throughout through your nose
- Ensure you utilise your full weight distribution of the foot
- Inhaling find your heel, exhale find your forefoot
- Push your knees forward as your hips bends and have a 60% heel weight distribution with a 40% forefoot weight distribution. As your hip extends or straightens, ensure you squash an orange and get your midfoot and forefoot to be doing 60% of the work while 40% of your weight is on your heel.

Phase 5 Exercise 1: Squat weight distribution with respiration

This movement will be very similar to your sit to stand exercises in phase 3. The difference now as we progress your load tolerance on your lower back is learning to relax more and to do less of the work, not by forcing your lower back to relax but rather allowing it to contribute BUT ONLY CONTRIBUTE its own fair share of the work and nothing more.

Stand with your feet shoulder width apart, eyes fixed on a spot, looking straight ahead if needs be.

Ensure your weight distribution is 50% of your weight on your left leg and 50% on your right leg with the majority of that pressure on the midfoot on each foot.

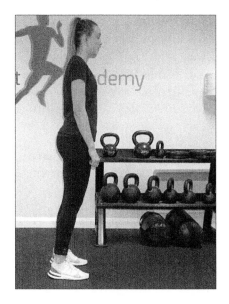

Ensure that you start with the weight over your midfoot and not on your heels.

Now inhale gently as you sit your hips back or go to sit down onto a chair.

Push your knees forward at the same speed that your weight shifts back to your heels, synchronising these two movements with your breath as you inhale slowly.

Push your knees forward as your weight goes towards your heels while synchronising these movements with a slow steady inhalation through your nose.

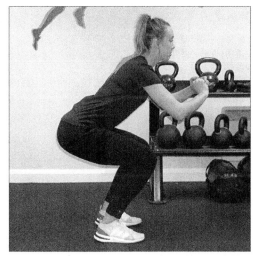

As you reach the end position, ideally as your weight is shifting back to the heels, without your toes lifting (ideally 60% of your weight on your heels, 40% on your mid to forefoot) and you just finish your inhalation, pause and then exhale slowly as you squash an orange through the midfoot and ascend upwards now changing the weight distribution of the foot to 60% on the mid to forefoot and 40% towards the back of the foot as you come back up to the start position.

Ensuring that you use the full foot, push the knees forward so you have to use the full foot. Breathing throughout the movement can be very useful to ensure that you use the whole body when doing squats.

The biggest mistake I see patients, even professional athletes, make when squatting is keeping their weight on their heels throughout the whole movement. This forces your lower back to react and contribute more to the movement. When you shift your weight on your foot, your hip will react more, meaning your lower back has to do less.

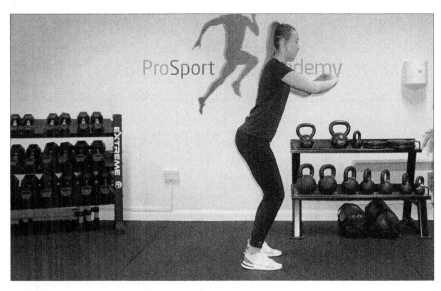

On the way back up, ensure you squash an orange through the midfoot and push the floor away as you ascend upwards.

This movement can now also be used when your pain sensation with sit to stands has been eliminated and the lower body is doing its fair share of the work so when you sit to stand, you can use this strategy without needing to tuck your chin to chest. But please ensure you are completely pain-free before going back to this option.

Phase 5 Exercise 2: Split squat weight distribution with respiration

This exercise is very similar to the previous exercise except your feet are not side by side but one in front of the other. This movement can be used in everyday life such as loading a dishwasher or picking something up off the floor.

Start with one foot slightly in front of the other so the big toe of the back leg is in line with the heel of the front leg.

Now start with 90% of your weight on the front leg and the back leg is just for balance essentially.

Start with your weight on the midfoot of the front leg.

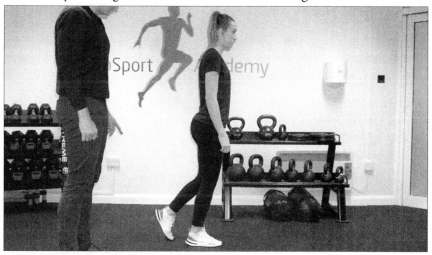

Start with the majority of the weight on the midfoot of your lead leg.

Inhale through the nose gently and slowly as you descend down to the floor, push your front leg's knee forward as your weight is distributed towards the heel, keeping 60% of the weight on the heel and 40% on the forefoot. Your back leg's heel can come off the floor if needs be and the knee is allowed to bend with the majority of the little weight that's on the back leg going through the toes.

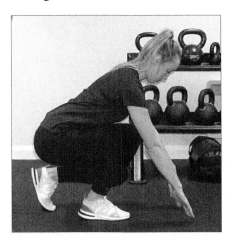

Push the right knee forward as the weight goes to the heel of the lead leg while also maintaining some pressure through the midfoot.

As you ascend upwards, the same rules apply as the squat, reverse the foot pressures and squash an orange through the midfoot so that 60% of your weight distribution is through the forefoot and 40% through the back of the lead foot.

Push through the midfoot on the way up throughout the movement as you ascend so the foot pressures reverse and the midfoot is doing more than the heel on the way upwards.

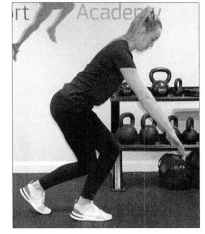

If you need to pick something up in everyday life, please ensure initially that you are squashing an orange through the lead foot to ensure that your legs are contributing to the load when lifting and you initiate the movement back up from the hip rather than leading with the head and hence the lower back. The intent first and foremost coming back up needs to be from the foot with the lower back finishing the movement rather than starting it.

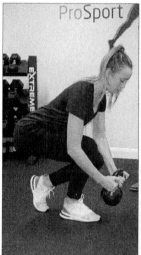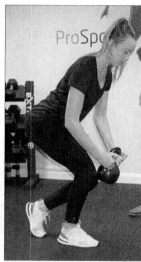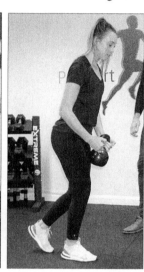

When picking items up during the day, please ensure the intent is always started at the foot and the lower back helps finish the movement rather than starting the movement.

Phase 5 Exercise 3: Lunge matrix with reaches

The final exercise I am including in phase 5 is the lunge matrix with reaches. This allows me to help you cover as many functional positions as possible without being completely specific to your needs.

The lunge matrix can be used instead of the split squat when you may only need to reach for something without having to bend all the way down. Hoovering would be one such activity where this movement pattern may be useful.

This movement will require your balance to be challenged further as you are now accepting weight from one leg to the other and with a small reach will further challenge your base of support. Remember from phase 4, when we reach in a direction, the foot will have to adapt to keep us balanced.

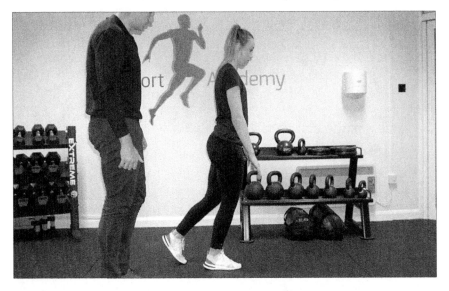

Notice the small step forward and the body weight is allowed to travel over the midfoot, similar to the weight distribution exercises from phase 3.

The key rule to remember with these exercises is that it needs to be a small step and a bigger reach to stimulate all the tissues and challenge you further. The biggest mistake you will make on this exercise is making too big a step forward so please be aware of this.

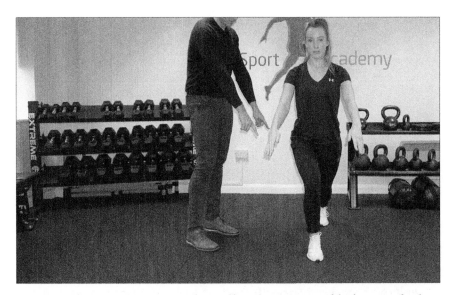

AVOID taking too big a step. This will make it impossible for your body weight to travel over your midfoot and not allow your base of support to be challenged in order to cause all the muscles in the lower body to react.

Start with both feet together and step forward no more than a foot in front of you. As your foot hits the floor, perhaps the heel touches the floor first and your knee is slightly soft; allow the rest of your body weight to follow over your foot stopping on the midfoot. Don't allow it to continue forward over the toes as the heel will raise and you will lose balance. This in itself can be the exercise to master first, before adding in the reach in the next step. This takes some of my patients a week to master.

To return to the start position, simply squash an orange through the midfoot and push into the floor in the opposite direction to where you want to get back to.

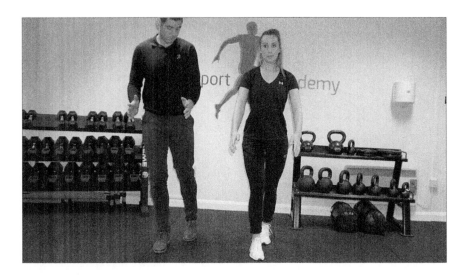

A small step with a soft knee allowing the body weight to pass over the midfoot without the heel coming off the floor.

Once you have mastered allowing your body weight to travel over your foot and accept your body weight on your midfoot we can think about adding in a reach.

This time as you step forward and your midfoot is just accepting the weight, reach your hands forwards as if reaching forward to pick a glass off the table; this will make it slightly easier to find your midfoot. Return to the start position by squashing an orange through the floor with your lead foot and returning to the start position.

Master the art of reaching just as your foot hits the floor to further challenge your base of support, and when you feel confident enough, progress to the next progressions.

Now instead of lunging straight ahead, you will lunge off to the side. Keeping your left foot facing 12 o'clock, you then twist your body so your right foot faces 3 o'clock as you lunge and accept your weight on your right midfoot. Again, add in the reach once you have mastered control of your body weight at this faster speed.

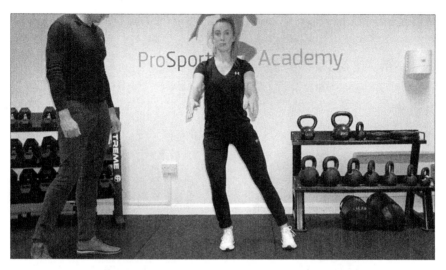

This time step sideways to 3 o'clock but ensure it is a small enough step that your body weight is allowed to travel sideways and over the midfoot again.

Finally we will challenge your base of support further and now twist your body and land your right foot to 4 or 5 o'clock as your mobility allows. Your left heel may need to come off the floor and your foot twist slightly – that is fine.

This time step and pivot to 4 or 5 o'clock. Again ensure it's a small step and allow your body weight to travel forwards so it's all over the midfoot of the right foot before you push back to the start position.

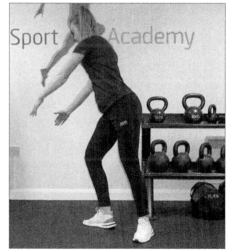

Again, accept the weight with your midfoot of the lead leg and once you are able to do this, add in the reach.

Now repeat the clock faces but with your right foot staying at 12 o'clock and your left foot reaching to 12 o'clock, 9 o'clock and 7 or 8 o'clock.

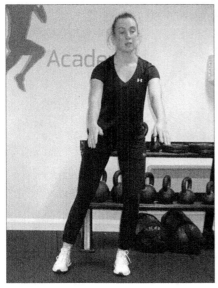 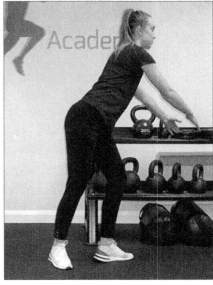

Small step to 9 o'clock allowing weight to travel sideways over the midfoot.

Small step to 7 o'clock ensuring all the weight travels over the left midfoot before pushing back again to the start position.

Perform three repetitions of each clock face ensuring good intent through the lead midfoot at all times.

If you struggle with one particular clock face to get your body weight over the midfoot, then you may gently have to push your knee forwards more as you land on the foot.

Mastering this lunge circuit will allow you to be able to twist and turn pain-free around a kitchen or workspace while allowing all the muscles of the lower body to do their fair share of work so the lower back does not have to do excessive work.

As I mentioned already, if you take too big a step forward then the lower back will have to react to keep your balance so please ensure you take a small step and allow your full body weight to pass over the midfoot of the lead leg. This is extremely important.

For demonstrations of these exercises, please visit **www. breathingmovinghealing.com**

So there you have phase 5. I have done my best to make these movements fit as many situations as possible and hopefully as you progress to phase 5 you have noticed positive changes in how you feel and move.

The reality is that everyone is different and so by this stage if you were a patient in my clinic, we would be making phase 5 specific to your needs and possibly progressing you further with increased speeds of movement and load tolerance on your body specific to your daily life. If there are still a few miles left for you before you reach your ideal destination then please reach out to me at our Facebook support group via **www.breathingmovinghealing. com** and I can do my best to put you in touch with a therapist trained specifically by me to implement a bespoke treatment plan for you for this phase. There is also a chance that we may need to go back and clean up some small things in phases 1-4 with you also so don't lose hope if your symptoms have not completely resolved by this stage if you have genuinely committed to and followed this programme accurately.

CHAPTER 10

What are the most common mistakes people make with the 'beating low back pain and sciatica system'?

Below are the most common mistakes people make when performing this progressive system. From my clinical experience, by identifying and correcting these mistakes, your chances of success will skyrocket and you will get to your ideal destination a whole lot quicker.

After you progress through this programme each week, please return to this chapter and review the common mistakes identified below. This will ensure that you do not make this mistake again.

Here are the biggest mistakes, in no particular order:

- Not focusing on your breath or slowing it down and ensuring it is light through the full repetitions while performing the task
- Not magnifying the feeling of 'safety' using your 'heartfelt' memory or feeling, in combination with a light breath with the bedtime belief restoration protocol
- Holding the breath while performing any of the movements
- Not distributing the weight through the feet in synchrony with the breath
- Not going super slow with the static weight distribution of the foot during the phase 4 exercises
- Not keeping the head still and the eyes focused on a spot while performing the static weight distribution of the foot exercises
- Not going super slow with the lunge and/or squat exercises initially and

pushing the knees gently forward to allow your midfoot to accept some of your body weight

- Holding the breath during the lunge and/or squat exercises
- Not distributing the weight efficiently through the full foot with the lunge and/or squat exercises
- Not 'squashing the orange' when pushing up from the chair, bed, squat or lunge movements.

This list is good to constantly refer back to as you progress through the programme. The more comfortable you feel with the exercises, the more likely you are to skip one of these steps and so it's always good to refresh your memory, as the attention to detail can make all the difference.

CHAPTER 11
Recap and refocus

Remember, there is no hocus pocus with any of these exercises or movements. We simply want all the different systems of your body – your respiratory system, your musculoskeletal system and your various neurological systems – to work in synchrony as they are supposed to, without you having to think about them.

At the start in phase 1 we obviously have to think about them in order to override some habits, both physical and mental, that you may have developed. As we get to phase 5, there is less and less conscious thought and more and more is happening subconsciously. There may still be more work to be done in phase 5 specific to your needs so please keep this in mind.

On a local level, we want the lower back to be able to do its job but we also want the mid back, ribcage muscles, and upper and lower body to also do their work and are working towards this from phases 1 to 5.

Now I want to quickly touch on some other topical issues that come up on back pain such as hands-on treatment.

Do I need a massage and hands-on treatment for my back pain?

This is a common question I get asked and there is mixed opinion with therapists lately. Hands-on treatment is OK in my opinion if used as part of a whole approach and part of the process. For example with us at ProSport Physiotherapy, if indicated you can expect to receive some hands-on treatment that may last a few minutes, that will be followed by some movement or movements that then reinforce the changes we are looking to make. What we would not want to do is get you to simply lie on the bed for half an hour and just do hands-on treatment. Why not? Remember the graph related to load tolerance in everyday life? Hands-on massage is very low on that graph and so in my opinion it's essential that your body is exposed to the relevant amount of loads it needs to tolerate in your everyday life. Sure, you might feel a bit looser leaving the treatment room, but what happens to most people when they go back into the real world and their mind and body are exposed to those loads again is that they go towards 'tension' and their bodies feel tight again or the unpleasant sensation may reappear.

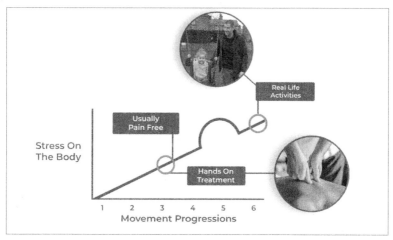

Notice how the demands placed on your body are far greater than what hands-on treatment can replicate. This is why, in my opinion, a lot of patients feel good leaving a treatment but the pain soon returns. It is essential that after the hands-on treatment, we continue to expose your body to the relevant amount of stress that it needs to tolerate in the real world.

Do I need any manipulation for my back pain?

Again this is a common question and indeed many people have got relief from manipulation from physiotherapists, chiropractors and osteopaths. What I would say is the same as with hands-on treatment: a manipulation can certainly bring about some changes in regards to muscle tone and how you feel straight away, but the key thing is giving your body an opportunity to tolerate loads it needs to tolerate on a daily basis and that's why the movement component is so important for long-lasting results.

Remember it is very easy to get rid of pain in the short term; it is a lot harder to keep that pain away and that is what you need to earn the right to progress through each load exposure without skipping steps, in my opinion.

What you might be thinking right now

What would it be like to have that freedom to wake up, get out of bed without pain, brush your teeth and have no limitations on doing the simple things in life pain-free?

But let's step back to reality for a moment, and address the elephant in the room. None of this is possible if we don't focus on understanding your story and linking it to your movement habits now, so that we prescribe the correct treatment and movement plan for you rather than just a set of glute or core exercises that 'might work' short term for most people. What we've done with this book is give you back as much movement options as possible that are very important for everybody in everyday life but we still need to have some specific movements and speeds of movements that are unique to your situation.

What you should be looking for in a therapist to help speed you along towards your ideal destination

Finally, I want to touch upon the type of healthcare professional, in my opinion, that you may require for support and guidance on your journey to your ideal destination if you choose to have one help you.

The most important thing, in my opinion, is that your therapist strives to understand your story, your past injuries, your past traumas or major events in your life and makes sense of how you are moving now as a result. Then it is critical that they understand exactly what you want to get back doing so they can design a bespoke treatment plan for you during phase 5 that follows a logical step-by-step load tolerance specific to your needs and bridges the gap from where you are now to where you want to be.

We've been very fortunate to have successfully implemented this system with patients of all ages from Huddersfield and surrounding areas. The ProSport Physiotherapy treatment approach is how you find the true cause of your back doing too much work for you with everyday movements.

When you implement this step-by-step system, you get CONSISTENT RESULTS that allow you to do the things in your life that are meaningful for you, enjoying conversations and activities with loved ones without the constant distraction of pain craving your attention. The result: a stress-free lifestyle.

If you need more help, we can help you further in two ways:

An Initial Assessment: for people who want to find the true cause of what's not doing its job and start treatment immediately to get the other body parts doing their jobs quickly.

A Discovery Session: for those people who are still a bit skeptical that we can help them, are wanting to get this problem solved and have a desire to get back to doing the things they love but are still a bit unsure.

Interested in either of those?

Then contact us at **www.prosportphysio.com**

The ProSport Physio Discovery Sessions are for purpose-driven people to solve their puzzle as to what body parts are not doing their job, so they can begin to experience the full joys of life again.

Remember, with the ProSport Physiotherapy Method, if you don't have the first step nailed, none of the others are a priority.

If you're just using the same exercises for 'managing' your symptoms without understanding what the true stressor actually is, then, unfortunately, you are just guessing.

Not truly understanding the true cause of your pain will unfortunately mean short-term results with the pain returning for a lot of people almost instantaneously.

THERE ARE TWO KINDS OF PEOPLE WE TREAT IN THE CLINIC:

1. Non-sporting people who just want to get back to everyday things in life pain-free

People who are looking to sit and watch TV without a constant ache, or lift their kids or grandkids again without having to think about bracing or holding their breath. People from West Yorkshire and surrounding areas who want to live life to the fullest, without second guessing if they will have to 'pay for it later'.

2. Professional and amateur sports people

We also use this exact same approach with professional and amateur sports people. While the outcome and destination will be slightly different, the process and step-by-step method is the same. This is because we see the person first and injury second.

YOU DON'T NEED ANOTHER MASSAGE, MANIPULATION, INJECTION OR SERIES OF PAINKILLERS

Or a whole load of new generic rehab or another Pilates class. You need to find the true stressor of your pain, specific to your body and your story.

You need a structured, common sense, logical step-by-step plan to identify the areas not doing their job and get them to help your low back so you can get back to doing the things in life that are meaningful to you.

- It's how Joanne overcame three years of chronic back pain, from the point where she could hardly move. After doing some research she came to the clinic and was able to take back control of her life. Joanne now lives free from pain and is back to doing her favourite things, keeping fit and enjoying life with her family.

- It is also how Steve, who had seen two consultants, had numerous injections and had been to other physios, osteopaths and chiropractors, got back to playing with his grandkids again after overcoming his seven-year-long back pain.

- Mark built his confidence up using this system and restored full movement so he could get onto his mountain bike again and take back control of his life.

- Victoria is a huge lover of running; she has progressed from barely being able to run to running whenever she feels she wants or needs to now.

- Rachel used running initially to help her with some mental health issues. When injury stopped her from running, it started to affect other parts of her life and relationships. Rachel followed this exact system and is now a published author, sharing her story.

- Anna decided to take up running but woke up one morning and her knee was very swollen and painful. By finding the true source of her knee problem and not just the symptoms we helped Anna overcome her knee problem. Anna now exercises five times a week, and is fitter than since her late teens.

- Putting his body to the limits and experiencing an injury just before a 115 mile race knocked Kevin's confidence, but coming to the clinic helped Kevin stay positive and he hoped not to be in any pain 50 miles in. Kevin completed the race in 46 hours without experiencing any pain using this approach.

The reality is that if you're ready to focus on what you truly want and are motivated to do so, you're likely only 6–10 sessions away from having the confidence to take on those complex tasks and jobs that you wouldn't dream of doing now.

If you follow phases 1–5 in this book, then you have given yourself a great shot at getting to the ideal destination. If you are completely pain-free now, after using just the movements and exercises in this book, then that would not surprise me one bit.

If you have noticed some really positive improvements but have a few more miles to go to get to the ideal destination, then that would not surprise me either because your pain and your story is unique to you. In this scenario, we may have some specific work to do with you during phase 5 to further reassure your nervous system and subconscious mind that you are safe, and that is fine too.

So there is no right or wrong if you still have symptoms but someone else doesn't. But there is help and hope available to get to that destination.

So, if you want those kinds of results like Joanne, Steve and others, and you feel you could benefit from this type of treatment, then book a discovery session to see if we are a good fit for you.

Live too far away?

While many people travel from all over the UK and other countries to see us, if you are reading this book and it's not feasible for you to travel to our clinic then that's completely understandable. The good news is I have personally trained over 250 therapists to date all over the world in this approach and I am sure we can put you in touch with someone closer to you. Please visit **www.breathingmovinghealing.com** and find the support section on the website to put you in good stead.

Are you a therapist reading this book interested in this approach?

We are also lucky to have many therapists who follow my work and the clinic's work. If you are a therapist interested in training in this approach then please visit **www.thegotophysio.com/mentorship** for more details.

Your next step

Well done on completing this book! Now your next step is even more important and that is making time and commitment to implementing this programme consistently on a daily basis. After the highs of the possibilities from this programme begin to quieten down in the next day or so, this is when the real hard work starts. Implement phases 1 and 2 throughout your day at any given opportunity. Phase 3 can be easily implemented at no great expense for 10+ hours of the day and give yourself 15 minutes before bed and when you wake to ensure your body is in 'rest and digest' to set yourself up for a great night's sleep or a great day ahead. Make 15 minutes in your day to focus on phase 4 while integrating your breathing and use the generic phase 5 movements at any opportunity throughout your day as your symptoms improve and your confidence grows.

Can you now see that this programme can and should be implemented in all areas of your life effortlessly with a little bit of focus and intent. The movements and exercises in this book are the key ingredients that most people overlook and use throughout their daily life. No fancy hocus pocus, just simple movements that you will do EXTRA-ordinarily over the coming weeks.

And remember if there's still a little bit to go on your journey, then be sure to visit **www.breathingmovinghealing.com** where we are always there to support you.

Be sure to email me on **dave@breathingmovinghealing.com** when you reach your ideal destination or major milestones on that journey. I love hearing about them and your story and journey. I look forward to receiving your emails. Remember to keep your attention on 'useful' thoughts, things and behaviours. Most importantly of all, this is your story and you are the one who will write the next few chapters in your life. How will they be?

Dave O'Sullivan is a Chartered Physiotherapist who has worked with England Rugby Union and Rugby League teams as well as numerous world-class athletes and organisations. Dave has a private physiotherapy clinic called ProSport Physiotherapy in Huddersfield that prides itself on offering non-sporting patients in Huddersfield and surrounding areas the exact same step-by-step system which he uses on a daily basis with professional athletes. Dave holds a degree in physiotherapy and also a master's degree in strength and conditioning.

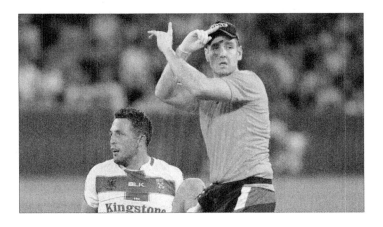

Notes

Printed in Great Britain
by Amazon

34227409R00088